Discover for yo...
the age-old key to
complete inner fulfillment

Each of us seeks a way of life that will bring
lasting happiness and peace of mind.
Yet far too often our tension-filled existence
prevents us from achieving spiritual
and physical fulfillment.

This book provides you with a key to the
timeless secrets of Meditation — the heart of
Yoga philosophy that has brought renewed
strength and serenity to millions everywhere.

Here, in clear prose and beautiful pictures,
you will find the meaning of Meditation and
the essential active and passive exercises for
relaxation, concentration and breathing.
Practiced daily, they can help you
gain self-mastery,
freedom from fears and restlessness,
a wonderful serenity in body and spirit.

Richard Hittleman's books,
classes and TV programs have enriched
the lives of millions of Americans.
This book — the essence of his teachings —
can do the same for you.

Bantam Books by Richard Hittleman
Ask your bookseller for the books you have missed

RICHARD HITTLEMAN'S

GUIDE TO YOGA MEDITATION

BANTAM BOOKS

TORONTO • NEW YORK • LONDON • SYDNEY • AUCKLAND

RICHARD HITTLEMAN'S
GUIDE TO YOGA MEDITATION

A Bantam Book / February 1969

2nd printing . . . . November 1969	8th printing . . . . June 1974
3rd printing . . . . . . October 1970	9th printing . . . . March 1975
4th printing . . . . May 1971	10th printing . . . . . . March 1976
5th printing . . . . March 1972	11th printing . . . . . February 1977
6th printing . . . . July 1972	12th printing . . . . June 1978
7th printing . . . . May 1973	13th printing . . . . March 1981

Cover and Inside Photographs by Al Weber

ISBN 0-553-14962-8

Published simultaneously in the United States and Canada

Bantam Books are published by Bantam Books, Inc. Its trademark, consisting of the words "Bantam Books" and the por-
trayal of a bantam, is Registered in U.S. Patent and Trademark
Office and in other countries. Marca Registrada. Bantam
Books, Inc., 666 Fifth Avenue, New York, New York 10103.

PRINTED IN THE UNITED STATES OF AMERICA

22 21 20 19 18 17 16 15

CONTENTS

To the eternal memory
of
Bhagavan Sri Ramana Maharshi

INTRODUCTION

The growing impact of Yoga upon Americans in all walks of life is one of the extraordinary phenomena of our time. Within a few short decades, this relatively obscure philosophy of the East has been successfully transplanted and nurtured upon the soil of American experience. Taken to heart by young and old alike, by students and housewives, by white-collar and blue-collar workers, it has proven beyond any doubt its effectiveness in bringing about a greater sense of physical, spiritual and emotional well-being.

When one examines the American "personality" (if indeed a people as variegated as ours can be said to possess a unified personality), it seems, at first glance, hardly likely that the Yoga physical and meditational practices should have elicited so strong and positive an effect on our nation. We are, after all, a practical and materialistic country, largely motivated by the pursuit of *things* rather than *ideas,* by pragmatic consequences rather than philosophic essences. Yet the deeply spiritual view of life which permeates Yoga has struck a responsive chord in the hearts and minds of Americans of all outlooks and occupations.

How can we account for this apparent contradiction? Why, at this stage in our nation's development, have so many here turned to a contemplative philosophy in their quest for a fuller and richer way of life?

As an instructor and writer on Yoga for more than twenty years, I have had the unusual opportunity to bring it before the attention of millions, and thereby to comprehend the reasons for its steadily growing popularity. With this knowledge and experience, I believe I can answer these questions in part by saying: Few people in the Western World are more subject to the anxieties, tensions, physical and mental ailments that are integral to a computerized, technological society. Hence, the attraction of Yoga — with its promise of relief from physical and spiritual malaise — for so many in our land.

While experimenting with certain methods of general instruction at Columbia University Teachers College, I discovered quite by accident that a bare minimum of Yoga practice performed by my fellow students and teachers (practice which at the time I all but forced upon them as part of an assigned project) produced some very dramatic results. The group with which I was working proved to me beyond a doubt that if a student were to devote only a brief period of time to certain Yoga physical and meditation practices — which I offered to this group in a highly condensed form — his ability to concentrate, assimilate and apply was remarkably increased. In a number of cases, the effects extended beyond the classroom and had far-reaching consequences of a very positive nature in all aspects of the students' lives. Until this time, Yoga, which I had been practicing in various forms from childhood, had been a very personal affair. But the results of these experiments with other people were so deeply stimulating and productive that after receiving my degree, I turned my full attention to the instruction of Yoga. I have been so involved for the past twenty years.

At the time that I began to teach professionally, the interest and understanding of Yoga, on the part of Americans, was virtually non-existent. Nothing could have had more of a "foreign" stigma. The Yogi (one who practices Yoga) was invariably confused with the Hindu *fakir* and was conceived of as the most weird, unearthly of all people. Declaring that "sitting on a bed of nails, walking on hot coals, serenading cobras and lapsing into deep hypnotic trances is not for me," the American summarily dismissed what he thought to be Yoga as irrelevant to his own life. Of course, it is now widely understood that the true Yogi is in direct opposition to the *fakir,* but twenty years ago the confusion between the two was practically universal.

To erase this erroneous image from the American mind and to convey the tremendous value that Yoga held, a number of instructors, including myself, began to present the Yoga science in a different light. Seeking to enable Americans to identify with Yoga, we emphasized the very great *physical* benefits to be derived from its posture and breathing exercises *(Hatha Yoga).* These exercises have been so perfectly designed to promote the healthy functioning of the organism and to develop certain latent potentialities, that it is almost impossible to perform them correctly for several weeks and *not* experience a profound sense of health and well-being. In addition, their therapeutic value in coping with many physical problems was well known to us. As we therefore proceeded to present Yoga primarily in a *physical* context, interest in it began to grow. We found that Americans could indeed identify more readily with the *physical*—with exercise, sports, health, etc. The Yoga exercises (*asanas*) subsequently imparted, in a manner much different from calisthenics, a high level of physical fitness to those who at this time undertook their practice. The word slowly spread.

Thus the *physical* properties of Yoga were stressed in this era of instruction, the supposition on the part of teachers being: If the student were drawn into the physical practice the health benefits would be so pronounced that he would then desire to learn more of the *philosophy* and to practice the *meditation* techniques; these were, after all, the entire "essence" of the subject.

Although this theory was a valid one and increased the attraction, the number of Americans being *exposed* to Yoga as recently as 1960 was relatively very small. A few new books a year, an occasional magazine article or newspaper interview with an instructor were the extent of the exposure — and this was usually undertaken by the media from the viewpoint of the bizarre or strange. But then, as we shall see, certain events transpired which focused national attention on Yoga and introduced its practice to millions of Americans.

Classes which I taught personally during the 1940's and 50's were well attended and I had the opportunity to work closely with many hundreds of students. From this experience I became more and more convinced of the efficacy of introducing Yoga to the greatest possible number of Americans. My belief was that this would have a most positive impact on all levels of the society. Those problems which seemed to most plague the nation: tension, anxiety, emotional instability, the need for a sensible plan of physical fitness, the search for more real values, the quest for self-realization could all be dealt with in such a *practical* manner through brief periods of Yoga practice!

In 1961 I conceived of Yoga instruction through a television series to reach the population *en masse*. The reactions of various producers in New York and Los Angeles to whom I presented this idea would provide the reader with a good many belly laughs. Needless to say, the producers did not trample one another in an effort to gain rights to the series. Eventually, however, I contacted an organization which *did* have the necessary vision and which *did* eventually make *Yoga For Health* a television reality. The programs are currently in their seventh year. While the series was still in the planning stages, one of the production company's executives said to me, "Your presentation is fine and we think the exercises are excellent. But couldn't you call them anything other than 'Yoga'?" This was in 1961. The "foreign" stigma was still in full effect. This year (1968) while discussing the format for a television "special" which would deal solely with the various aspects of Yoga in the United States, a network official said to me, "But couldn't you allow your hair to grow long and wear some robes? You just don't look like a Hindu!" Thus, within one decade, Yoga in America would appear to have come full circle.

The current younger generation, having both the need and the time to seek a way of life other than that offered by the "establishment", has been an important factor in generating Yogic interest, especially in the past few years. It is natural that in its quest for certain basic truths and wisdom this generation would be led to examine the culture of the Orient. The current phenomenal popularity in the Western World of oriental music, art and philosophy — including Zen Buddhism, Taoism and Yoga is the result. Visiting Hindus have established schools and *ashrams;* meditation groups are flourishing everywhere. The interest in self-discovery and self-realization is at an all time peak in the United States — and rightly so. Our society, having over-developed itself on the material level, now feels the absolute necessity of achieving a balance by developing its spiritual resources. This being the case, one need have no fear that the current Yogic interest is a "fad". A number of younger people who have professed an interest in Yoga, meditation, chanting, etc., simply to conform to the "in" group will, of course, eventually turn to other things, as will many of the people whose only objective is to lose a few inches from their waists. But no person who has been genuinely attracted, who has caught even a glimpse of what Yoga has to offer, can ever truly abandon its pursuit. Also, we must understand that Yoga, like nature, needs and seeks no help in perpetuation. Both are eternal; together they fulfill all needs of the individual. To think of Yoga as a "fad" — in the sense that interest in it will soon pale and it will gradually fade away — is out of the question.

Through my television programs I have had the privilege of instructing a great many Americans in Yoga. But because of certain obvious limitations that are imposed by this medium I have been able to devote only a minimum of time to the discussion of Yoga philosophy and meditation. I am therefore grateful for the opportunity afforded me by this book to present a concise interpretation of both these subjects which I know, from many years of teaching experience, can be of inestimable value to the reader. What is true of the practice of physical Yoga is equally true of Yoga meditation: It is impossible to undertake the serious application of the principles set forth in these pages and *not* experience a profound positive change in *all* aspects of one's life.

Richard L. Hittleman
Carmel, California, 1968

USING
THIS
BOOK

This book is designed to point the way toward a particular and unique experience. Section I — the philosophical section — is meant to impart to the reader more of a "feeling" of the Yogic wisdom than to appeal to his intellect. Each of the concepts and techniques discussed in this section is usually treated in very great detail, often requiring many volumes, in the classical writings of Yogic scholars. However, for most Americans who desire a practical working knowledge of the *principles* of Yoga, these detailed expositions, which even in the various English translations are replete with hundreds of Sanskrit terms, are usually discouraging.

Therefore, the elaborate philosophical details of the original works are here reduced to what I believe constitute their "essence." As such, the reader is advised to carefully reflect upon and digest each chapter before proceeding to the next. Each meditation technique should be experimented with for at least one week so that the reader can derive a "feeling" of it and determine what value it holds for him, personally. When preparing to practice any of the meditation exercises of Section I, it is necessary to refer also to Sections II and III.

Because the philosophic principles are highly condensed, the various chapters will acquire a new and expanding meaning each time they are read. Therefore, if the reader's interest in Yoga is serious, these chapters should be reread regularly. But remember: one cannot read the philosophy and discount the meditation; the two are inseparable.

Yoga is an experience, not a system of thought; it is to be lived, not intellectually analyzed. To achieve this, meditation is indispensable!

SECTION I

YOGA PHILOSOPHY AND MEDITATION

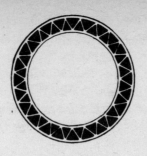

CHAPTER 1.

THE GREAT RIDDLE
OF
THE SELF

Who are you? A strange question! But you really do not know where you came from. You are a temporary resident in this life. You do not know where you are going when you leave. If you will pause to reflect, you will discover that you really know very little about who you *really* are; not your name, or your address, or your family, or your business, or your social activities — these are all things *about* you. But if all these things were removed and you had nothing external by which you could describe yourself, then who would you be?

"Know Thyself" is the classical philosophical advice offered by both Eastern and Western "masters" throughout the centuries, for in this "self" lies the whole answer to the riddle of life and death and to subsequent peace of mind and spirit. But who is this Self? How does one go in search of it? Where is it hiding? What sort of directions are necessary to find it, and if it *is* found, how does one learn to "know" it?

YOGA is man's oldest known method of scientifically dealing with the great riddle of the self. It prescribes first that we take a real close-up look at the hidden aspects of this self. For example, we continually use the word "I." But how well do we know this "I" — his opinions, his beliefs, his likes and dislikes? Could it be possible that the real YOU may have absolutely nothing to do with the I who decides what he likes and dislikes, what he is going to do and not do, etc.? This is certainly an unusual concept, because we generally worship our I and attempt to cater to him in every way, giving him what he wants and nourishing his beliefs, his likes, his desires. It comes as a shock to be told that the I is actually a stranger in our house who has gradually taken over our lives and now runs things entirely his own way!

In the study of Yoga we learn that we have not nearly the understanding of the I that we may like to think we have ("I know myself very well") and that we further, have almost no control over what the I now is or what it may become. In other words, the self or I controls the true YOU and tells you what to do. Since we do not understand how this self has tricked us, we blindly obey its commands. *All of our so-called "problems" of life have arisen through our ignorance of the way in which the self operates and these problems are dissolved only when we are able to realize the true nature of our self.* Yoga, in its philosophical aspect, can be considered as a series of techniques for investigation which, when seriously applied, will help to reveal the truth about the self and the role which it plays in our existence. You will be very much surprised at what you are going to find out through this investigation!

Investigation into the "I" of the Body

The essence of Yoga practice is contained in the techniques known as *concentration* and *meditation.* These may be said to originate with Yoga. In its elementary form, concentration takes the form of *observation.* The first exercise of our study is called *Observation of the Body.* How well do you know the "I" of your body? How much control do you have of him?

The Yoga physical exercises you will be learning in the pages to come will provide you with wonderful means of relieving tension and relaxing. In conjunction with the stretching postures you will be awakening a great deal of sleeping energy. It is essential that you conserve this energy. Have you ever realized that your life-force *(prana)* may be burned up and wasted without your knowing it? It is essential to conserve and store this life-force in your body for purposes of self-development.

The major causes of dissipation of life-force are: (a) nervous habits, (b) association with negative persons, (c) misuse of your senses, (d) idle talk. Look about you anywhere and you will see people tapping their feet, twiddling their fingers, twisting their mouths, chewing gum, chain-smoking, pacing restlessly, indulging helplessly in dozens of nervous habits and useless actions which merely waste the life-force so that it is not available when needed. Much of this is, of course, the expression of fear, anxiety, anger and other unhealthy mental and emotional conditions.

People who practice the self-control which Yoga teaches impart a feeling of controlled energy. They are efficient; they go about their work with a minimum of effort, with no wasted energy and few unnecessary movements. They seem to get straight to the point and are always ready to take quick, forceful action when they have to. People whose energies are being wasted, or whose life-force is being sapped from their physical, emotional or mental bodies, are generally worn-out without knowing why; they tire easily and cannot count on having sufficient energy available when they need it. Such people are blown about by life like a leaf in the wind, without stability or certainty, and for them life is a never-ending series of frustrations, problems and tragedies.

You must now learn to relax in each of your activities. Make every move count. Take a lesson from the cat who so well represents potential energy. Notice how he moves, stretches, relaxes. He looks disinterested and almost lazy, but let the mouse run by and the cat pounces upon him with one swift, forceful movement. The cat wastes no energy. He can teach you a great deal about conservation.

To learn more about your wasteful actions, learn to observe yourself at sudden, frequent, unexpected intervals during the day. Stop what you are doing and look at yourself in action. You will be surprised at how you catch yourself wasting energy through unconscious nervous habits and tensed muscles. You can make a game of this. Whenever you can remember to do so, observe your body in action and notice where and how you are tense. Let your mind run quickly over your entire body, beginning from your toes and working upward. Gently and calmly order all of the strained muscles and all tense areas which are making no direct contribution to what you are doing, to RELAX! Notice whether you are making useless, wasteful movements in your activities. If so, send a message to the areas involved to *relax and not to repeat these movements*. You must actually give this order because you are dealing with something which you will find is very much like a child; it will do things its own way and push you as far as possible until it is corrected.

Your body must be disciplined like a child, calmly but forcefully. You are, in fact, re-educating your body and as the various areas are convinced that you are serious (just like the child), they will begin to obey. Simply observing that a muscle is tense is not enough in the beginning; *you must give it the order to relax* and you may have to repeat this order frequently over a period of some time before the "child" learns to respond. But as it realizes that you *are* serious, it will respond. Remember that it takes a lot of your energy to hold a muscle tensed or in a strained manner, to tap your fingers or feet, or to chew gum for several hours. If you are doing these things, especially unconsciously, you are certain to be losing vital life-force.

Another important loss of life-force occurs when you are in the company of certain people. Many persons, not having sufficient life-force in their own organisms, draw on the vitality of those around them. Unless you know how to prevent this life-force from leaving your body (which you will learn as you practice these techniques), you will feel exhausted, depressed and negative after being in the company of these people. If you know which people have this effect on you, try to avoid their company as much as possible. Associate whenever you can with people who have as much or more life-force than yourself and who leave you with an elevated, positive feeling.

Idle chatter is another way in which many people continually use up their life-force. We tend to talk a great deal and actually say very little. Much of this conversation is because we are afraid of sitting still, afraid of silence. Notice how many people you know have come to depend constantly on their radios, phonographs and television sets to prevent silence and to keep their senses occupied. Many persons are also concerned with what others will think of them if they are not "social" and do not keep up an endless stream of meaningless small talk. But remember that here again, talking requires great energy, especially idle chatter. The reason why monks and nuns of all religions and orders take vows of silence is so that they may conserve their life-force and help to quiet the restlessness of the body and mind.

Further, to conserve life-force, you should begin to pay attention to your emotional body. (The word "body" is used because the emotional and mental aspects of your organism have a subtle form and structure). The emotional body should be as quiet and calm as possible. This entails, among other things, not becoming involved with forms of amusements which drain the energies from your emotional body. Television programs, movies, newspapers, and magazines that are preoccupied with lust, violence, murder, sin, sex, etc., force you to devote your thoughts and attention to them and in many cases to actually "live" them. That is why several hours of television viewing will often leave you limp and exhausted.

It takes energy to think and act on all of these things and such energy is a poor investment, since all you do is pass the precious hours of your life and feed your mind with negative thought forms. There is very little return for this investment. Most of our forms of "entertainment" do not relax us and do not stimulate us positively. They pulverize our nervous systems and make us more tense and emotionally strained than ever. Do not be tricked into giving your precious time and energy to these things.

In summary: *Any activity which leaves you physically or emotionally drained and exhausted is to be absolutely avoided whenever possible.*

Practice of these self-observation techniques along with the physical postures for relieving tension (See Section II) will enable you to experience wonderful new vitality as well as an elevated and calm state of mind. As you gradually reach this state of body and mind, the negative situations of life will have less and less power to sap your life-force.

CHAPTER 2

IN QUEST
OF
HAPPINESS

We all want to be happy, to get the most out of life. We strive continually with all of our resources for fulfillment, satisfaction, contentment and peace of mind and soul. And yet you have only to look around you to realize that unhappiness and discontent are everywhere and that money, success and fame do not, in the final analysis, bring one closer to the real peace and understanding of life which you seek.

Many of us know full well that there seems to be something radically wrong with our "values" and we can speak with intellectual authority on the social, financial, domestic and political reasons for our having been swept up in the mad merry-go-round of our present life. There are those who do not know that they are on the merry-go-round. There are those who know it rather vaguely but do not care. There are those who know it and *do* care and *who want to get off.*

It is the last category of people with whom Yoga is concerned. Many of the people in this last category who are weary of their restlessness, dissatisfaction and frustration will often turn, in desperation, to anything which seems to promise relief. Mental sciences, the various "positive thinking" schools, spiritualism, the occult sciences, hypnosis, narcotics are but some of the paths chosen.

But we find, sooner or later, that none of these things can provide us with the ultimate peace that we really seek, because these things are all substitutes; they attempt to treat the symptoms, not the cause; they temporarily numb the pain, but do not get at the *cause* of the pain.

The increasing indulgence in various drugs prevalent among the younger people of our society is a case in point of the correct objective with the incorrect means. Their need to transcend the ordinary mind, to search out their true natures, to escape the highly questtionable economic and social demands of the society, to experience euphoria and an elevation of the spirit, are all understandable and commendable.

But drugs are dangerous. Their real danger

is not only physical (from the Yogic point of view, even the mildest stimulant used regularly, will result in an eventual deterioration of the nervous system and inhibit the natural awakening of the life-force) but *spiritual*. That is, the change of consciousness which manifests in varying degrees according to the drug used becomes so desirable, indeed, so essential to the user, that his dependence upon it gradually becomes permanent.

When the user is "on," he feels that he catches a glimpse of reality, that he is in tune with his true nature. When the effects of the drug have worn off and he is "down," the unreality of what he erroneously believes to be the "mundane" world becomes intolerable. Therefore he must revert more and more to the use of drugs. He no longer wishes to question why it is that if he has indeed experienced "reality," he must continue to come "down." He no longer wants to be told that *real* beauty lies only in the "mundane" world he is attempting to escape.

The crux of the matter is this: What is actually perceived by the user when he is "on" is not reality; it is a *counterfeit* of reality. It is close to the real thing but it is not genuine. Some teachers have described this situation as "a knocking on the back door of heaven." The spiritual danger is, then, that the more the drugs are used, the more counterfeit reality which is experienced and the less inclined (and the less able) the user becomes to undertake those physical, emotional and mental disciplines necessary to experience a *genuine awakening*. The spiritual realization which the drug-user believes is drawing closer and closer is, in the long view, actually receding.

The user of drugs, in an attempt to escape the "merry-go-round," is not different, in the final analysis, from the various other methods named above. Again, the symptoms not the causes are treated; the pain is numbed, not dissolved. Therefore, suffering must continue to return in one form or another throughout one's life. If we would have real peace of mind, body and spirit, we must pierce through directly to the heart of the matter, to the *cause* of our dissatisfaction.

Ordinary and Universal Mind

From Yoga we learn that there are different levels of consciousness. We are all familiar with the fact that there is a sub-conscious and a conscious mind. These two states of consciousness make up what we will call our "ordinary" or "every-day" mind. In addition to these, Yoga explains that there is also a higher or *super* consciousness which we will refer to as *Universal Mind*. All of our problems, confusion and suffering in life stem from the fact that we do not understand the nature of our "ordinary" mind and are unaware that we continually possess the power of the Universal Mind.

We do not perceive how our ordinary mind has taken over and runs our lives. It tries to serve in many capacities for which it is not equipped — which are actually reserved only for our higher consciousness. As such, we find ourselves continually in the most perplexing circumstances and beset by problems for which there seem to be no solutions.

Because most of us are unaware of the existence of the Universal Mind (or being aware of it, we do not know how to use it), we have come to rely upon, and indeed even worship, the dictates of our ordinary mind, since we believe that such dictates are always in our best interests. We have come to believe the incredible fantasies which the ordinary mind invents for us.

Twenty-four hours a day this ordinary mind operates, filling us with outrageous notions which require all of our energies and attention. We faithfully undertake to do everything it tells us, because it has hypnotized us into believing that if we listen to it and follow where it presumes to lead us, it will eventually provide us with the happiness and peace which we are seeking.

But the ordinary mind is actually very similar to a machine. We can well compare it to one of those fantastic computers about which we read and hear so much these days. It selects and processes data and then interprets this data in a very particular way and a very *limited* one. Our great error lies in believing that this machine-like ordinary mind is *unlimited* and that it is perfectly competent to gather in all of the necessary facts and all of the information that is needed to make the right judgments and to deal effectively with any situation which arises.

And so we listen to what the machine-mind tells us, because we have faith in its ultimate ability to lead us down the path of peace and fulfillment. We chase after its empty promises, hoping to complete successfully a business deal, build a house, buy a car, meet that person, travel to this country, attend that school, etc., all with the hope that doing these things will finally make us content.

And as the months pass and we may indeed gain many of the things which our ordinary mind has told us to seek, we find a whole host of new desires and "necessities" have arisen and that having satisfied the old desires has not brought us a bit closer to real peace and contentment. We are just as far from true security as ever. But the fact that we have not fulfilled ourselves leads us to fix the blame on any and every conceivable "outside" circumstance, from "destiny" and "fate" to just plain "bad luck," and we fail to realize that it is the misunderstood workings of our ordinary mind that bring us time and again to the point of frustration.

The Wheel of Life

Thus we come to learn that the usual method

of seeking happiness through the mechanism of the ordinary mind is like looking for the pot of gold at the end of the rainbow. We know there can be no "end of the rainbow" because what we see of it is merely part of a circle. So it is that our ordinary mind forces us to travel around and around in a great circle, promising us always that the pot of gold lies just beyond. But this pot of gold which we can call our "goals" and "objectives" in life recedes before us like the horizon.

In our Yoga study we use the symbol of a wheel which we call the "wheel of life" to indicate how we are imprisoned in the vicious circle of attempting to satisfy our endless desires. Upon this wheel, each of us must pass through all of the possible conditions of human existence, alternating between opposites, as day follows night, unable to realize the peace which we desire and to drink the waters that will truly satisfy out thirst.

Attempting, therefore, to find peace through the channels of the ordinary mind is like trying to put out a fire with oil. We believe falsely that we may find such peace by satisfying our desires and set out to do so. But every time we believe that we are getting close to having arranged our lives, our jobs, our friendships, our possessions so that we can at last be happy and secure, we find that conditions have changed, that people are different, and that new problems have arisen which force us to begin and continue the whole deceiving process again.

We find ourselves like the circus performer who sets many dishes spinning on the end of poles and then dashes madly back and forth among them in a frantic effort to keep them revolving. What actually happens to us is that the nature of the ordinary, machine-like mind is so preoccupied, so distracted by the things of everyday life, of day-to-day existence, it is unable to convey to us the true nature of the world and of ourselves in relation to it.

We erroneously seek happiness and contentment by attaching ourselves to objects, persons and conditions of the world. If we can only awaken from the trance, the hypnotic spell under which the ordinary mind perpetually keeps us, we will begin to understand how we have allowed the machine to take over, the peculiar manner in which we have fallen asleep to the reality of our own existence!

Now this is not to imply that the ordinary mind is to be done away with. On the contrary, it is indispensable to cope with the *mechanical* and *technical* problems of our life. Being like a machine, the ordinary mind has access to statistics and is therefore able to tell us how to handle our business, how much money we have in the bank, what we would like to have for dinner, how to drive our car, what appointments we have for the day, etc. But when the facts take over and keep on feeding themselves to us without our being able to stop them, then they may lull us to sleep and we lose our true identity, which is that of the Universal Mind.

Imagine a television set on which the switch is broken so that you cannot turn it off. You sit and watch the programs endlessly until there comes a time when you forget that there ever was an "off" switch. That is what has happened in the case of our ordinary minds. We let the thoughts run on endlessly, hour after hour, day after day, year after year, giving them our full attention and energy until we forget that they are simply facts, statistics, being played over and over like a phonograph record.

We will, therefore, not minimize the importance of our factual, ordinary mind and of its so-called "logical" thinking process. But we must realize and always try to remember that what we know through this ordinary mind is only a tiny fraction of what there is to *know* and that *real knowledge and real wisdom* do not lie within the scope of the ordinary mind. Such *wisdom,* also known as *truth,* can only be apprehended with Universal Mind. Let us make this simple summary: *truth and wisdom* ARE *Universal Mind.*

Our ordinary mind has more or less convinced us that we can solve our problems through its "logic" and "reason" and that there are no situations or circumstances in which the logical thinking of our ordinary mind is not the most important and desirable factor. In our society today, we truly worship "logic" as a god and quickly dismiss as "illogical," "impractical" or "unreasonable" anything which lies outside the limited thinking methods to which we have grown accustomed.

Thus our "machine" rejects almost anything it cannot explore through the aid of the senses and think about logically. And even though the methods of the ordinary mind have failed time and again to provide us with the one ultimate security which we all seek —PEACE— we continue to place the blame not upon our blind obedience to this limited mind-machine, but on imaginary *external circumstances* "beyond our control."

The Tragedy of the "Self"

The fact is that we have never understood our problems in their correct perspective. We do not realize that the ordinary mind creates our problems and then, in its own good time, attempts to solve them. It makes us believe that the problems are on the "outside" and that we can only cope with such problems through the resources of the ordinary mind. The ordinary mind, being a machine, has but one function: It creates and then goes about attempting to solve problems! It enjoys this game and will continue to play it as long as you allow it to do so, throughout your entire life if it can. It is not concerned that you are suffering in many areas because of its games. You will come to understand through the meditation techniques that *you are not your ordinary mind* and that it has not nearly the importance which we attach to it.

The entire concept of "internal" (within) and "external" (without) and of each of us existing as a separate individual apart and different from our fellow man is an illusion — a dream — of the ordinary mind. This is one of its games. This ordinary mind, along with the senses and the emotions (which it uses as its cohorts to help play its games), has succeeded in creating the idea of a separate "ego" so that each of us has the impression that he has, and is, a separate self; that without it he would lose his identity and in some way or other would cease to exist. But nothing could be further from the TRUTH. Indeed, the exact opposite is true, as we shall see.

The real tragedy of the dream of the self is that it prevents us from knowing our true nature, that of the Universal Mind. In many of us the higher consciousness tries to make its presence felt, but the ordinary mind would have us look upon these "mystical" experiences with great suspicion. It makes us reject anything that does not fit into its habitual patterns of thought and analysis.

So, not understanding the nature of either the ordinary mind or Universal Mind, we live our lives, forever victims, forever suffering (in one form or another) and unfulfilled. The ordinary mind, together with the emotions and senses, plays endless games of intrigue within the framework of the self, and as long as we have no understanding or control of these things, we must remain their victims. The point is: We have never been shown how to become the master instead of the slave; how to relegate the ordinary mind to its proper place, which is *to take orders and not to give them.*

Our efforts to understand our self, to find peace of mind and spirit, to lead richer, more integrated lives, to realize the purpose of our existence, can never be successful if we seek these things with our ordinary mind, regardless of what philosophy, mind-science or self-improvement methods we try. But these efforts are successful the very moment we are able to truly realize the eternal presence of the Universal Mind and that we can allow it more and more to take over our lives. Indeed, it is the ultimate surrendering of our life, the "letting go" of our ego, which constitutes liberation and enlightenment *(nirvana, moksha, samadhi.)*

In this study, we must do much more than make vague, abstract statements about "love," "peace," "soul," "spirit," "brotherhood," and God. These are empty phrases which the ordinary mind cannot possibly comprehend. There is no *"understanding"* of love, God, etc.; they can only be *experienced. Realization of the Universal Mind and the experience of love, brotherhood, peace and truth are the same thing.*

You can begin to conceive the difficulty in

attempting to explain what the state of realization of the Universal Mind is like, for in order to do so, the explanation must be directed toward the ordinary mind, which is the very thing we are attempting to transcend. No intellectual understanding of the Universal Mind enables one to escape the tentacles of ordinary mind. The ordinary mind will think about the Universal Mind in its own circumscribed "logical" manner, which it envisions as a loss of identity, or associates Universal Mind with becoming a "good" or "better" person. But none of these ideas are *true*. You cannot, therefore, attempt to reason about and understand the super-consciousness. You can only experience it!

Active and Passive Meditation

The investigation of the "self," of which we have spoken before, is undertaken through the various techniques of meditation. Meditation may be *active* or *passive*. That is, it may be practiced in the midst of any and all of your daily activities, in which case it is *active*, or it may be practiced in privacy and solitude when you temporarily have physically withdrawn yourself from the world of activity for a designated period of time each day. In the latter case it is *passive*.

To continue our investigation of the self, let us next use the technique of *observation of the ordinary mind*. Just as we previously tried to catch the body where it is tense and unnecessarily strained, draining our vital energies, we will now attempt to learn how the ordinary mind is needlessly sapping our life-force and how, by allowing it to run wild, without control, it binds us each day more and more to the wheel of empty promises and endless desires.

At frequent intervals during the day, whenever you can remember to do so, observe your mind. Notice if it has been concentrated on what you are doing, helping you to do it with the maximum efficiency and least expenditure of time and energy, or if it is wandering, continually distracted and filled with thoughts that have no bearing on your work.

Persons who cannot concentrate their minds on the point of their work generally prove inefficient. They waste time and energy and the quality of what they do is poor. Knowing how to concentrate will open up new faculties of the mind and give you an insight into how to accomplish what you must with a minimum of effort.

Also, during your leisure hours, notice if your mind is cluttered with idle day-dreams, wishful thinking, repetitive thoughts of the past and fantasies of the future. Such workings of the ordinary mind sap our life-force and lend substance and reality to the illusionary way in which we see the world and ourselves in relation to it. If you use the above methods of suddenly, unexpectedly getting the "feel" of your ordinary mind, of observing the thoughts which are passing through it at various times of the day, you will become very aware of how much these thoughts include useless concern, false anxiety and foolish daydreaming.

Remember that it requires a great amount of life-force to *think* and that much of what floats through your mind during the day, beyond your notice or control, is simply not worth this expenditure of vital energy. The ordinary mind tends to become like a phonograph record that plays over and over; if you do not change this record, you waste your precious life listening to the same old tunes again and again. Soon you forget that the record *can* be changed or the phonograph turned off and you are lulled to sleep by its hypnotic repetition.

Whenever you catch the machine-like, ordinary mind playing the record, distracting you, filling you with useless thoughts which consume your valuable time and vital energy, *order it to stop!* Tell it in no uncertain terms that you are not interested in these superfluous, meaningless thoughts and that you do not want them to arise again. If you will issue this order whenever you observe the ordinary mind involved in its antics, it will soon stop forcing your attention upon these things.

But you must be on your guard and persevere with the practice of this observation technique. Use your ordinary mind when necessary for your activities, but when you are finished, you should turn it off. Be aware that the machine does not have to run continually. It can and should be rested.

Through this observation practice you will, more and more, be able to quiet the restlessness of your ordinary mind and greatly conserve your life-force. As the ordinary mind is stilled, one is able to become increasingly aware of the presence of the Universal Mind. Therefore, the physical and mental observation techniques which we have termed "active meditation" become extremely meaningful.

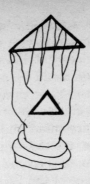

CHAPTER 3.

THE THREE BODIES: KEY TO SPIRITUAL UNITY

We know that we have a "physical" body; but we will now learn also of the "emotional" and the "mental" bodies. These actually *exist* in the sense that they are composed of matter. However, this matter is far more refined than the physical body and consequently the emotional and mental bodies are known as the "subtle" bodies. It is important to understand that the emotional and mental bodies, being composed of matter, are subject to the laws which govern matter. These laws are, however, of a higher order, since the matter which they govern is of a highly refined nature. These higher laws are known in the Western World as the study of "metaphysics." If one understands the metaphysics of the subtle bodies, he can learn how to gain control of them.

We find that in most of us these three bodies are disorganized. The body, mind and emotions each seem to go their separate ways and wish to be independent of the others. They are not integrated and do not act together as a single unit. As such, you have a continual feeling of confusion, of an inner tension, since the physical body pulls one way with its desires and needs, the emotions pull a different way, craving their own satisfactions. The mind runs in still another direction, demanding that it be given full attention. Under such circumstances how can one be expected to function efficiently, be single-pointed in his objective and gain any degree of spiritual insight?

The Objective of Yoga

At this point of our study we can define the word "Yoga" as "integration." Other definitions may be given as "unity" or "joining together." These are all more or less the same. In Yoga, you attempt to integrate or join these separate bodies and this integration enables you to function under full power, producing a great "awakening" of your latent faculties. The awakening destroys the illusion or dream of your separate "ego" which is the thing that keeps one a perpetual slave to worry, fear, anxiety and insecurity. All of the philosophy and techniques both physical and mental are for the purpose of accomplishing this integration.

In working for integration, you attempt to achieve what is known as "one-pointedness." That is, you can work with one of your three bodies, temporarily making the others subservient to it so that only the one with which you are working receives purposeful attention; the others do not have the opportunity to continually interfere and pull you in different directions. When, for example, you are working with the physical postures, you do not allow your mind or your emotions to pull you away and distract your attention. The body reigns supreme during the practice of the exercises. When you work with your mind (in meditation) you allow no interference from the physical or emotional bodies.

Since in this course of study we practice with both body and mind, our progress can be accelerated. The physical postures should automatically call for your full attention and their very practice quiets and relaxes the mind as well as the body. That is why, if you do the postures correctly, *the physical practice becomes a form of active meditation!*

Another way of discussing Yoga is to employ the word *unity.* In working toward integration, we attempt always to be aware that *all objects, thoughts — everything that is manifest in the entire universe — both seen and unseen, known and unknown — spring from one source and re-*

turn to this source. Behind everything is one supreme intelligence — Universal Mind. But this truth is generally very difficult to grasp when you are subject to the many distinctions continually made in the everyday world. Our ordinary observations are based on noting the *differences* between things. Society intentionally emphasizes these differences (politically, economically, socially, etc.) so that we grow farther and farther away from truly understanding the unifying principle behind all worldly phenomena.

We tend to believe that what we see about us is not only *real* but *permanent.* This is not true. Through the Yogic study we become acutely aware that everything is in a state of continual flux and change, of continually *becoming.* We may contemplate, as one of our meditation techniques, the transitory nature of all objects, ideas and conditions. When the ordinary mind realizes that its own true nature is *continual change* and that nothing which the senses perceive has any true permanence, it becomes ripe to abandon its fruitless chase after the illusion of satisfaction, fulfillment and security through attaching itself to things and conditions of the world.

Thus the student of Yoga learns to gradually control his senses (because of the peace which results from this control) and he is able more and more to turn his mind *inward.* By examining his senses and *understanding,* in the most profound sense of the word, the manner in which they function, he can trace them to their point of origin. At this point of origin he experiences *unity* and he realizes how the apparent differences which he has observed in the "external" world are actually the result of the way in which the senses function.

As one becomes aware of this principle of unity, of oneness, he finds that the various aspects of his organism, the three bodies, begin to integrate. One can look for an unparalleled feeling of peace as this happens, for you have the sense of true security rather than being like the leaf in the wind which is helplessly blown about in every direction. But regardless of how fully one may understand the problems of the ordinary mind and its infinite delusions, this understanding with the intellect can never by itself quiet the organism or achieve the unity and integration of which we have spoken. To accomplish this we must use the specific techniques of meditation; integration is an *experience*, not an intellectual theory.

We have stated that the student of Yoga traces the origin of his senses. A great river may have many tributaries and you can find this main stream by following any of the tributaries back to its point of origin. So it is that the senses perceive many things which appear different and separate but actually arise from a common source. When you are able to perceive that you too have come from, are sustained by, and return to this source, you realize your supreme identity. The river of your individual self merges with the ocean of Universal Mind and Yoga is achieved!

Now it has already been pointed out that we have very little control over the ordinary mind; it is continually in motion. If you can learn to suspend its incessant movement for only a brief interval, you begin to realize how this ordinary mind keeps you in a state of perpetual confusion, uncertainty and insecurity. The situation is similar to what transpires in watching a movie. You allow yourself to be deceived by the apparent movement taking place on the screen. Really, however, you know all the time that this is an illusion but you permit yourself to be "hypnotized" by the illusion. If the film were slowed down or suddenly stopped on one frame, you would "snap out" of the trance and become fully aware of the nature of the illusion. Similarly, if you can bring your mind to rest upon a single point, even for a very short period of time, you can begin to awaken from the hypnosis of its continual motion.

We have so far learned two very important methods of *active* meditation: (1) observation of the movement of the body; (2) observation of the thoughts of the ordinary mind. These are techniques which can be practiced at any and all times of the day. Now we are ready for the first of the *passive* techniques of meditation.

Passive meditation may in itself take several forms. One of these is known as *concentration*, or *one-pointedness*. You know from experience that it is generally somewhat difficult to concentrate. It seems to take a special effort to put your mind on a particular subject or idea and keep it from its usual countless wanderings and distractions. But concentration as we practice it in the study of Yoga becomes one of the most relaxing and enjoyable activities of the day.

First of all, the object of our concentration is interesting and pleasurable. Secondly, this type of concentration renews the energies of the organism; lastly, even the slightest degree of success with the concentration techniques will begin to make you aware of the higher consciousness, of Universal Mind. As this occurs many of the seemingly hopeless problems of everyday life dissolve and they do so naturally, effortlessly and what is often called "miraculously."

The Techniques of Concentration

In concentration we use the various *senses* as our instruments. We choose one with which to work and the others become subservient to it as explained above. Since *sight* is the most developed of our physical senses, we shall begin concentration with a technique which makes use of the *eye*. In the beginning we will have two kinds of concentration with the eye: *external* and *internal*.

For *external concentration* take any object that pleases your eyes: one that you enjoy looking at. It might be a flower, a vase, a figure, an interesting symbol or design. Place this object where you can look at it easily without eye strain. Sit in a comfortable cross-legged posture as explained below. Now fix your eyes on the object you have chosen and keep them there.

Naturally, for the gaze to remain fixed on the object is no problem, but allowing no other thought (other than the contemplation of the object) to distract you is difficult. To accomplish this one-pointedness of observing and contemplating only the chosen object, use the following aids: Notice the various aspects of the object, its color, its shape, its use, etc. In short, let your mind dwell only on the various aspects of the object and do not allow it to wander or be distracted by other thoughts.

It will be most revealing to discover how often your mind will leave the object during the three minutes prescribed for this concentration technique. When you begin to realize how rapidly and continually your mind must be moving all through the day and night, you will understand how it is able to keep you disorganized, in a state of confusion and uncertainty, and how little control you really have of it.

Each time you find that your mind has wandered from the object, you must return it, gently but firmly. At first you may not be able to focus your thoughts and hold them

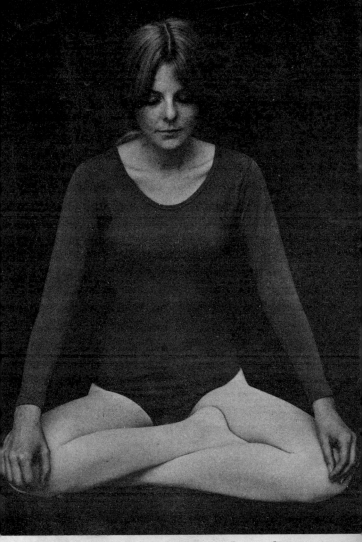

FIG. 1 *The simple Cross-Legged posture. The ankles are crossed and the legs drawn in as far as possible. Wrists rest on the knees; eyelids lowered.*

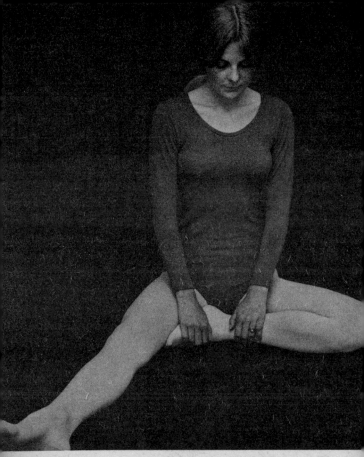

FIG. 2 *Preparation for the Half-Lotus. The left heel has been placed as close in as possible.*

FIG. 3 *The completed Half-Lotus. The right leg has been placed to rest either on the left thigh or in the cleft of the folded left leg. Wrists rest on the knees with index fingers firmly touching the second joint of the thumbs. Eyelids are lowered.*

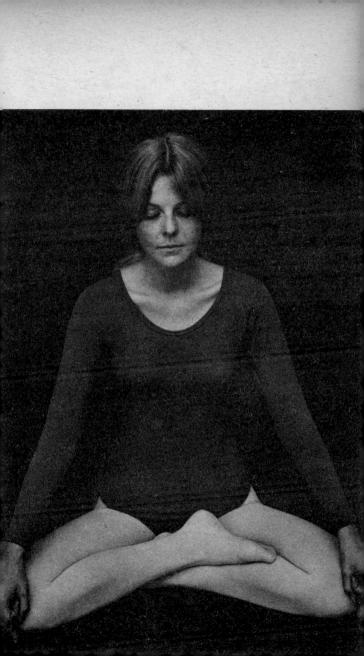

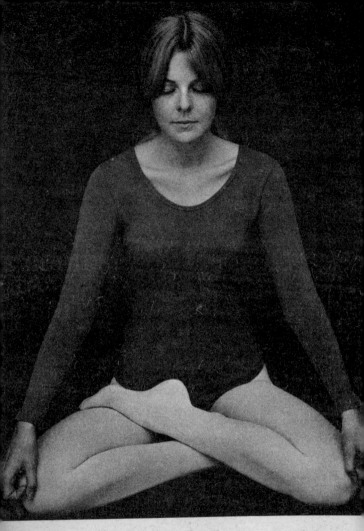

FIG. 4 *The Half-Lotus with the legs re-versed. The left foot rests on top of the right thigh or in the cleft of the right leg. The student must determine which position of the Half-Lotus is the more comfortable.*

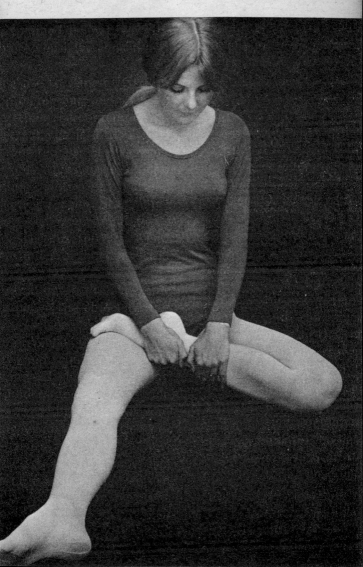

FIG. 5 *Preparation for the Full-Lotus. Either foot is placed to rest on top of the opposite thigh.*

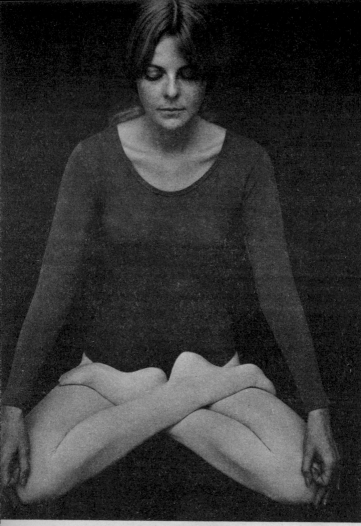

FIG. 6 *The completed Full-Lotus. Both feet rest on the thighs. Palms may face either up or down. Eyelids are lowered.*

Any one of the positions depicted in Figs. 1, 3, 4 or 6 are acceptable for the various meditation exercises.

for more than only 10 to 15 seconds on the given point! But with continued practice, that is, bringing your mind back each time it is distracted, you will gradually train it to remain for increasing periods of time on a single object.

Do not scold your mind or become angry when you find that it has tricked you again and again and always carries you away from the thing you want to observe. Simply return it to the object and make a mental note, saying to the thought which is distracting you, "I am busy now and I cannot listen to you at this time." Words to this effect will slowly but surely convince your ordinary mind of the necessity of one-pointedness. You will find that when you gain some success with this technique, your everyday activities, business, social and domestic, can be handled with more assurance, more ease, more efficiency. This is because you are gradually becoming "integrated," in the deepest sense of the word, and you can do more things in less time and do them well.

We have spoken previously of the fact that the training of the body can be compared to the disciplining of a spoiled child. It has had its way for a long time and it expects to go on having its way. When you attempt to change its patterns it fights, it rebels. The same is true of the mind, only much more so. When you attempt to change the stubborn habits of your ordinary mind, it too will fight and its chief weapon is to make you weary and lazy so that you will not want to practice. Do not allow it to continue having its way. It is time now that you became the master in your own house.

Simply sitting down quietly at least once each day for just *three minutes* and fixing your gaze upon a pleasant object, contemplating it without distraction, will automatically begin the process of integration within you! To measure the three minutes you may use a timepiece, stop watch, or simply try to judge the time. Do not glance continually at your watch. You must try to be aware the moment your mind begins to wander and return it at once. Otherwise you will allow many valuable seconds to elapse without realizing that you are off on a tangent.

There is ingenious deception and trickery in the ordinary mind which you will come to realize through this concentration technique. This type of concentration may also be practiced in an *active* manner. That is, at any time of the day when you find yourself with a few spare minutes, while relaxing, riding in the bus, waiting in an office, fix your eyes on a single point (you can simply lower them to look at the floor) and attempt to hold your mind on this point. This practice will be of much greater value to you than the meaningless, futile thoughts which generally occupy the ordinary mind while riding, walking, waiting. Remember: *No one can strengthen, control and concentrate your mind for you. This you must do yourself.* Begin now and resolve to no longer be the slave of your thoughts!

Candle Concentration

Here is an additional and very ancient technique that you will find fascinating and valuable. It is known as "candle concentration" and is another way of using the sense of sight for concentration, this time not only externally but *internally* as well. This is also a most relaxing technique.

Sit in the cross-legged posture and place a lighted candle approximately three feet from you. Gaze directly into the flame of the candle (blinking as necessary) for approximately two minutes. Then close your eyes and press the palms of your hands lightly against your eyes. When you close your eyes, you will retain the image of the flame. Concentrate on that image and do not let the flame wander or disappear. If it should disappear, bring it back by simply looking for it (with your eyes closed all the time). Fix your mind completely on the image of flame and let no other thoughts distract you. Keep the palms pressed against the closed eyes for an additional two minutes, making approximately four minutes in all. Each time the flame disappears or your mind wanders, bring it back. Soon you will be able to hold the image of the flame steady with your eyes closed. There is a great restfulness that results from candle concentration.

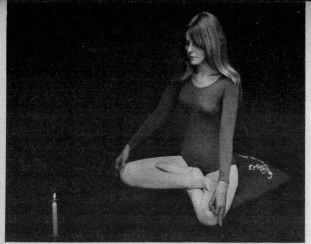

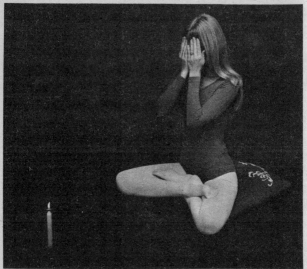

FIG. 7 *The gaze is fixed and held on the lighted candle for approximately 2 minutes.*

FIG. 8 *The eyes are palmed and the image of the flame retained for approximately 2 minutes.*

62

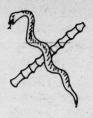

CHAPTER 4

AWAKENING
THE
"SLEEPING" MAN

Yoga classifies individuals as "sleeping," "awakened," or "enlightened." The "sleeping" man is not aware that he is using only a fraction of his great potential power. He plods his way through life in a conditioned hypnotic state as a prisoner of his ordinary mind and his five senses. He may be "successful" in all of the ways of the world. He may appear to be a man who is "happy" and "satisfied" in the ordinary sense of the words. And yet, if he has not been able to perceive what lies beyond his senses and has been unable to transcend his ordinary mind, the Yogi will say that this man is "asleep."

The "awakened" man realizes that he is not using his great reservoir of potential resources. He knows instinctively that there are powerful forces available to him if he can but learn how to utilize them. The "awakened" man is intuitively involved in attempting to contact and use his dormant power.

The "enlightened" man is the ultimate objective of Yoga practice. He has aroused his latent forces and controls them; he has transcended his ordinary mind and is able to integrate himself with the Universal Mind. As such, he is no longer affected by the fears, anxieties and weaknesses of people still in bondage to these things. Only the "enlightened" man understands the true nature of the universe and his relation to it. He retains the ever-present realization that he is not separate from the universe but an intrinsic part of it. He erects his universe and because of this, he knows eternal peace.

Yoga is concerned with you as an "awakened" individual. The "sleeping" man has no true interest in the higher consciousness; the "enlightened" man has achieved his goal and his studies take a different form — one which transcends our understanding at present. Your interest in Yoga is an indication that you have reached the stage of "awakening." This did not happen suddenly, nor is it an accident. There has been a methodical evolvement; a slow, systematic stimulation of your higher consciousness during a period of many incarnations. If your interest is strongly drawn toward Yoga, you have probably been engaged in its study or that of related subjects in previous incarnations.

You have a great responsibility not only to yourself, but to your fellow man to advance your development as far as possible and to help awaken the higher consciousness of those persons who are ripe for such knowledge. Relatively speaking, only a very small percentage of the world's population is "awakened" at any given time in the course of world history. That is why when you mention Yoga to many of your friends and relatives, they are completely at a loss to understand your interest in this study. However, it is most significant to note that the interest of the Western World in Yoga is more prevalent than at any time in recent history.

How does a "sleeping" man awaken? As stated above, this is not an accident. He has spent an untold number of lifetimes passing through the initial stages of the lower consciousness. (We will discuss *incarnation* in detail later.) Through sheer weariness with trying to satisfy his insatiable desires does he begin to look elsewhere for fulfillment. It requires an astronomical period of time until he is ready to admit to himself that he is indeed subject to fears of every description, including death; that his anxieties regarding everyday living never cease; that he seems unable to gain real control of his emotions and his mental faculties; that living, in its ordinary sense, holds no true happiness, security or peace.

Only when he is absolutely convinced of the truth of these things does it occur to him that he has been searching for his fulfillment and peace in the wrong places and using the wrong instruments. It is at this point in his evolution that the sleeping wisdom within him is stirred and he experiences an awakening.

Once awakened, he cannot go back to sleep. Usually there is a great inner struggle as one treads the winding path between the states of "awakening" and "enlightenment." Progress on this path is dependent on many factors and one develops in accordance with how seriously he applies himself. Spiritual evolution for the awakened man can consume a myriad of lifetimes or it can culminate in "enlightenment" within a relatively short period of time. It is largely a question of how important real peace and true security are to the individual.

There is the story of the master (guru) and his student who were sitting at the edge of a river and discussing the practice necessary to achieve enlightenment. Suddenly the master grasped his student about the neck and held his head beneath the water. The student struggled to release himself but the master held him firmly. Finally the master pulled his head from the water and released him. The student gulped air into his lungs.

Then the master said, "When I held you under, what was the uppermost thing in your mind?" "Air, air," gasped the student. "Exactly so must you crave enlightenment," stated the master.

It is very difficult for us in the midst of our everyday activities to realize the illusion in which we are continually immersed. That is why you must try to remind yourself at every opportunity that your ordinary mind is presenting you with a very partial and obscured view of everything that happens to you. What is before you, the present situation which is being interpreted for you through your senses and ordinary mind, is a type of mirage.

We have spoken of the motion picture projector which projects an illusionary picture upon a screen. We know as we look at the screen that this picture is an illusion. In reality the characters are not alive upon the screen, nor do they actually move. It is the film that is moving. But we are contented for the sake of watching the picture to *pretend* that the events depicted for us upon the screen are real.

Similarly, in a very peculiar manner, do we pretend that what happens to us in the course of our everyday activities is real. But gradually, as the "awakening" becomes more intense, we realize that the ordinary mind and the senses have constructed a giant house of cards in the way we see ourselves and the world about us. If you pull away one of the bottom cards, the entire structure collapses. An objective of Yoga practice is to gently and methodically pull away the bottom cards in order to reveal the weakness of the structure.

As you contact the higher consciousness, Universal Mind, you become more and more aware that you have imprisoned yourself in the darkness of a tiny, suffocating cell. This cell has become familiar and your eyes have grown accustomed to the dark, to the way in which you see yourself and the so-called "external" world. You have forgotten that outside the cell is the world of light, of freedom.

The cell is not *apart* or outside of this world of light; it is a tiny particle *within* it! By the same token your ordinary mind is simply a particle within the Universal Mind. Thus Yoga does not ask you to give up your ordinary mind, but simply to realize that it is only a tiny fraction, a tool of the Universal Mind.

How do you have this realization? How do you come to know that you *are* Universal Mind? For one thing, it begins to occur automatically as you practice the meditation techniques. The ordinary mind begins to dissolve into the Universal Mind and this permits the higher consciousness to take over, relieving you of much of the terrible burden that the ordinary mind is helpless to cope with. An excellent way to accelerate this evolution is to instill into yourself an awareness of your higher consciousness — to manifest a sudden elevation of your entire being just by your will — so that you instinctively look beyond that erroneous and limited view of the ordinary mind to the Universal Mind. Try it right now: *Will* yourself into an expanded state of consciousness. This is your birthright.

These techniques of "awareness" must be applied to all of your activities and the situations in which you find yourself in the everyday world. *Transcend the situation.* It is as though you have simply *asked* or *willed* your higher consciousness to take over your life, and whenever you feel that it has deserted you, *simply will it back.* Each time you thus *will* your higher consciousness into play, you are allowing the light of the Universal Mind to dispel more of the darkness of the ordinary mind; each time you utilize this technique, whether it be once a month or several times a day, you grow.

You will find yourself functioning more efficiently in every way as the higher consciousness responds to your needs. Your life appears to go on as usual outwardly, but inwardly a great change, a tremendous *expansion*, takes place. The enlightened man is the result of the ultimate expansion; he has grasped the infinite wisdom of the Universal Mind; he has realized *that man is spirit!*

Concentration with the Ear

Let us now use another of the senses for

purposes of concentration. We shall use our sense of sound and direct our entire attention upon it. As with the eyes, there can be two forms of concentration: *external* and *internal*.

For external concentration, choose a particular sound upon which to focus your attention. This can be a sound of nature such as the singing of a bird, a sound of water, a river, the ocean, the wind. Again, the mind is directed toward this sound and not allowed to wander. All of the other senses are temporarily suspended in their functioning. When you find that your mind has wandered, you must bring it back again and again to the sound, gently but firmly. Always give a mental order to the distracting thought which says in effect, "I am busy now and do not want to be disturbed."

A practical exercise is to listen to a recorded selection of music for approximately five minutes. The music selected should be interesting, something which you enjoy hearing. Sit in a cross-legged position and lower your eyes (do not close them, since this is associated with sleep; just lower them so that a slit of light can pass through). Listen very carefully to the music and begin to lose the thought of "Here I am listening to this music." If you are properly concentrated, there will be no thoughts at all.

Do not let yourself become sleepy. Try not to let the music conjure up pictures or other images, because these will distract you. *At-*

tempt to make yourself an instrument through which the music may flow. As your ego, your ordinary mind, your self, your "I" becomes immersed in the depths of the sound, you will find your consciousness expanding. You are no longer hearing and understanding and analyzing in the usual limited way, but you are able to encompass the full significance of SOUND! This realization is beyond anything which the ordinary mind can conceive and is, of course, beyond description.

The *internal* method of concentration with the ear is more subtle and requires intensive concentration. Sitting in a quiet place, either indoors or outdoors, you attempt to *hear the sound within your own ear!* Did you know there was such a sound always present? This demands a complete withdrawal from the external world and is a fascinating challenge. See if you can locate this internal sound which is similar to the sound made by the ocean waves striking the shore. Hold your attention upon this sound for three minutes. Naturally the moment any thought or outward disturbance arises, you will lose the sound and you must then bring it back.

Concentration with the ear, either internal or external, should be done for three to five minutes. This is a *passive,* not an *active,* form of concentration. That is, you must be alone and very quiet to achieve success with the sound technique. It is tremendously relaxing and refreshing.

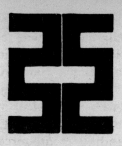

CHAPTER 5.

LIFE FORCE: THE SUSTAINING POWER OF THE UNIVERSE

An ancient Yoga text proclaims: "Life is in the breath!" This is a fact which none of us will dispute, since we well know that our existence is dependent upon continuous breathing. We know that it is possible to exist for extended periods of time without food, water or sleep; but without air, death is certain to result within a matter of minutes. However, it is much more than just this that the Yogi implies with the above proverb. He is speaking of a most profound matter in which the "breath" is but one manifestation of the life-force.

The science of Yoga can become extremely intricate. In this book it is assumed that you are interested in learning the information and techniques which are absolutely practical and can be immediately applied. Therefore, the many Sanskrit terms and phrases which would require volumes to explain and whose practical value is questionable have been eliminated. The concept and understanding of *life-force,* however, is indispensable, since all of the Yoga physical and mental exercises which you learn are involved with accumulating, storing and using life-force. We must, therefore, have a good idea of this subtle element and how to work with it.

Many centuries ago, Yogis, who were extremely analytical and who possessed what we would call "highly developed extra-sensory perception," were fascinated by the phenomenon of breathing. Their investigations led them beyond the physiological aspects of breathing, i.e., beyond the structure of the lungs, the circulation of the blood and the gases which comprise the air.

They observed that in addition to the oxygen which the blood was assimilating from the air taken into the lungs, there was another more subtle element being absorbed by the organism. They eventually recognized this element as a force which was present in all things manifest in the universe, and they named it with the Sanskrit word *prana,* which, as it is translated here, becomes "life-force." Another translation could be "pure, absolute energy." The Yogis formulated laws concerning the workings of the subtle life-force, not only within the physical body, but within all matter.

And so, since very remote times, the Yogis knew the entire universe, from the most dense compound of mineral elements, throughout the plant and animal kingdoms, to the complex organism of the most sensitive species of human beings — and beyond — as being permeated with this life-force. It pervades every atom of our bodies. It is not the atom itself, but the core and soul of the atom which imparts to it its direction and its ability to function. It is the intelligence and force of the atom.

Through this life-force is fashioned all forms and structures of matter; it activates each atom, from those which comprise the most dense mineral substances through all of the degrees of increasingly complex organisms. It makes possible all organic functions both conscious and subconscious. It is the medium through which the process of creating, sustaining and destroying is carried out.

It is an acknowledged fact that we are able to hear and see only within a limited range of both the sound and the sight scale. We know that there are sounds, for example, whose pitch vibrations are at frequencies above and below our range, so that they are inaudible to the human ear. This limitation also applies to our other senses, including faculties of sight, smell, taste and touch. These limited senses confine us within a world of three dimensions. The serious practice of Yoga enables one to transcend these limitations in varying degrees, the outcome of which is to perceive that not a single particle of matter in the entire universe can remain still, stationary, for one moment.

Everything is incessantly in motion, continually changing and forever *becoming* something different than it was at the preceding moment. Thus, all things, including those which ordinarily seem to be the most inanimate and dense — the wall, the table, the bricks and stones — are in reality permeated with life-force and shimmering, or *vibrating*. We begin to realize that what we formerly considered as devoid of life is simply vibrating more slowly on what might be called a different wave length, but that it too is a manifestation of the life-force.

Indeed, life-force is present in all things, gross and subtle, in all matter and in all thought, and you live in your present form only as long as the life-force exists in certain proportions within your body. When the life-force leaves your organism, it ceases to function. This is the state of "death" as far as the physical body is concerned. Hindu *fakirs* (not to be confused with Yogis) who allow themselves to be buried for long periods of time without access to air know the secret of retaining the life-force within the body.

In the study of Yoga, the more life-force which you are able to utilize, the more physical energy and vitality, the more mental alertness and the more *awareness* you will come to possess. Persons who radiate vitality and energy and who have a "magnetic" personality are in possession of an abundance of life-force. You know, for example, that a radio station which operates with 50,000 watts is going to be much more powerful than one which uses only 5,000 watts. The former station can be picked up for many times the distance of the latter. Similarly, when you add life-force and energy to that which you now have, you are certain to become much more powerful; your vibrations are increased; your physical and mental organisms are greatly elevated and you thus come in contact with the higher planes of thought and action.

All of the techniques learned in Yoga are concerned primarily with (1) releasing a great amount of life-force which is already within you but which is sleeping and needs to be stimulated and aroused, and with (2) accumulating additional prana from external sources. Life-force is derived from food, water, sleep, sunshine and certain other elements. Air, however, is the most immediate, accessible *and powerful form of life-force!* That is why it is so important to learn and practice the wonderful methods through which we can extract increased life-force from the air as presented to us in the various forms of Yogic breathing.

Diseases certainly will result when the life-force, for one reason or another, is lowered or reduced in a particular area of the body. The Yogi will actually diagnose an illness in terms of a "lack of life-force." The Yogi contends that all of the drugs, therapy, surgery, etc., that are administered to the patient are actually an attempt on the part of the physician to stimulate the action of the life-force so that *healing* may occur. There is no doubt that many persons do indeed shorten their lives due to the reduction in life-force and that this is very often caused by improper breathing! You can realize the great value of correctly learning and practicing the price-less breathing techniques which are presented to you in the study of Yoga.

Conserving and Observing the Life-Force

We have discussed a number of important ways in which you may be wasting and losing your life-force. You should continue to re-read these sections and definitely put the advice offered into practice. It is wasteful to learn and practice all of the wonderful physical exercises of gathering increased life-force if you are wasting or losing this energy in the ways indicated.

Now the fact that the physical eye cannot

actually "see" the life-force does not alter the truth of its presence in all things and that it is responsible for maintaining your very life. You cannot see the force of gravity and yet you know it is continually exerting its influence upon every physical object on the face of the earth. Gravity is a form of life-force. And just as you know that gravity exists, although you cannot see it, so will you come to know of the existence of life-force, not only within yourself, but in all things.

As you continue to practice your Yoga physical exercises and meditation techniques, you will come more and more not only to "feel" the reality of this force, but to know how to direct it to various points in your own body as well as to distant parts of the world. You should be able to use this cosmic force for the health and development of your self as well as others. Persons who are successfully practicing the occult sciences have mastered certain aspects of the life-force. Although in the study of Yoga we are not interested in the "powers" of the occult sciences, we will also work to gain control of this force, but solely for purposes of spiritual development.

Concentration with the Breath

In *passive* concentration, we have previously employed two of our senses: sight and sound. Now we will use a more subtle element which requires increased powers of concentration. Remember that our objective in all of these techniques is the same: the quieting of the ordinary mind. It is the frantic behavior of the ordinary mind that is the great obstruction to the perception of the Universal Mind. We will now breathe with the movements of the Yoga Complete Breath and attempt to *observe* the breath as it is inhaled, retained and exhaled. This is one of the most powerful techniques for the quieting of the mind.

In classical Yoga texts the breath is spoken of as the "string which controls the kite." The kite in this analogy is the mind and the breath is the string. As the breath moves, so moves the mind. If your breathing is short and rapid, your mind will work nervously, agitatedly. If your breathing is erratic, your mind must be disturbed and anxious. But if your breathing is long, slow, smooth and even, the wildly racing, mechanical nature of your mind will become tranquil and peaceful!

The breath is the link between body and mind; it is the stepping off place from the "physical" to the "mental." Actually, the body and mind are but two parts of the same thing; they differ only in density, vibrations and certain other qualities of form and function. As you carefully observe your breathing you will begin to perceive that point at which the so-called "physical" changes into what is known as "mental."

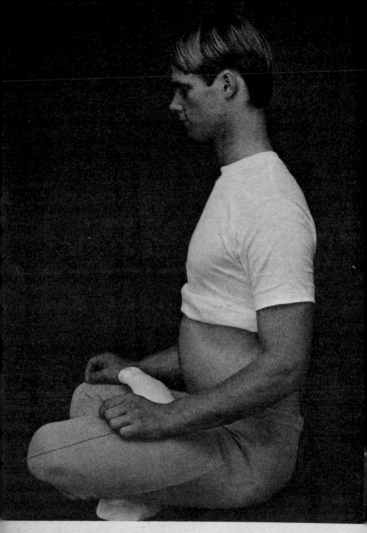

FIG. 9 *The abdominal area is distended during the first part of the Complete Breath.*

FIG. 10 *The chest is expanded as far as possible during the second part of the Complete Breath.*

To perform meditation with the breath, sit comfortably on your mat in a cross-legged posture. Lower your eyelids until only a slit of light remains. Remember: *Do not close your eyes completely*. Next, begin the move-

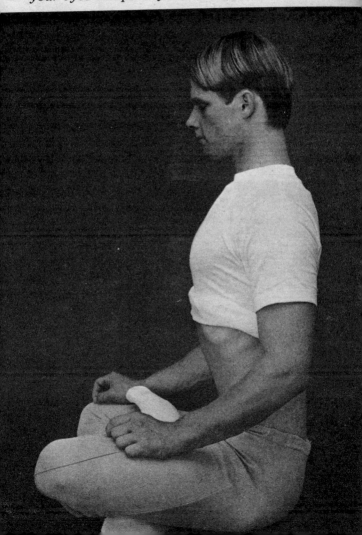

ments of the Complete Breath. Slowly perform a deep exhalation and then begin the inhalation. Distend your abdomen (simply push out with the abdominal muscles) as you slowly and quietly inhale through the nose. (Figure 9). Continuing the slow, smooth inhalation (do not stop the inhalation) fill the lungs completely and expand the chest as much as possible (Figure 10). Without pause, slowly and quietly exhale, allowing the body to return to the beginning position. Without pause, begin the slow, quiet inhalation and repeat the body movements.

Observe the air entering your nostrils. Follow it with great concentration during the entire inhalation. Try to see where it comes from and where it is going as it enters the body. Observe what is happening to you as you exhale. Do not allow the breath to become lost. Keep your attention on it. If and when the mind should be distracted, simply bring it back as we have discussed previously in connection with the other concentration techniques.

Perform this technique for approximately three minutes. You will begin to learn wonderful, fascinating things about the subtle elements and forces within you and all around you that you may have taken for granted throughout the years. The passage from the Bible which tells us that God "breathed life into the nostrils of man" is most interesting in this connection. The breath is a primary clue to your identity as Universal Mind!

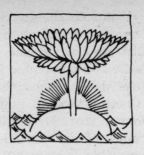

CHAPTER 6.

HOW THE YOGI
SEES
THE UNIVERSE

The Yogic viewpoint of the Universe is of a much greater scope than anything with which the Western World is familiar. Whereas we have been led to accept the theory that man has somehow evolved from a more primitive creature and that civilization may be approximately 7,000 years old, the Yogi would comment on the former statement as "absurd" and the latter statement as "yesterday."

There has been no beginning and there can be no ending to *eternity*. The word "eternal" is impossible for the ordinary mind to understand, because to comprehend something, this mind must be given information pertaining to *qualities*, i.e., shape, color, size, form, etc. Only when the ordinary mind has this type of information can it make judgments about the thing at hand. But what is "eternal" has no qualities. It is beyond shape, color, size, form, etc. It is true that qualities reflect an aspect of the eternal; that is, the eternal makes use of qualities as an agent, but the agent is not the eternal.

Consequently, the ordinary mind can have no true understanding of the eternal. It simply is not equipped to function in an eternal dimension. A child in the third grade might be able to solve problems in addition, but he is not equipped for differential calculus. Similarly, the ordinary mind is very limited in its ability to conceive what is meant by "eternal" or "Universal Mind." And even though we are awed by the incredible computing machines which the ordinary mind has been able to devise, *such mechanical ingenuity brings us not one iota closer to realization of the higher consciousness.* For this type of understanding, a much more refined instrument is necessary. We attempt to gain such refinement through the study of Yoga.

We know that there is "day" and there is "night." The cycle of day and night is completed each 24 hours. The Yogi speaks in terms of "day" and "night" concerning the existence of the universe. During the "day" of creation, everything is manifested; that is, all of the suns, planets, satellites, galaxies and everything which is upon these bodies, including man himself, *exists*. During the "night" of creation, all of these phenomena are withdrawn into a mathematical point and become suspended or "potential."

The creation dissolves during the "night" and lies asleep as a seed. When the "day" comes again, the universe is manifested and all things become *actual*. When the universe is in its state of existence, it is only a question of time (astronomic, of course) until it ceases to exist, and when it is non-existent or potential, it is only a question of time until it will exist again. There is no beginning and no ending to this cycle. It is eternal.

The period of this "day and night of creation" is very great as far as our concept of years is concerned. When we learn about the distance and sizes of the stars we are staggered, for it does indeed exceed the ability of most ordinary minds to comprehend such vastness. Similarly; is the day and night of creation counted in the billions of years. The period of time of the "day" is approximately equal to that of the "night." The Yogic texts state definite periods for the various cycles that are described.

Where does the individual stand in all this immensity? Well, if you think that you have an "ego" and that you are a separate "self," then you will find yourself lost amidst this concept. But if one is able to realize that he is not, in reality, an individual self, and that this self is truly an illusion, then he understands that he too is eternal and that he is not born and does not die. Thus one is not lost and all of the immensity is not a source of perplexity or anxiety. But again, the ordinary mind finds it impossible to follow this line of thought, because it must reason in terms of "beginning" and "ending." Thus it is limited and cannot conceive of eternity or what it is like *not* to have an ego; it is imbued with the thought that if something happens to the self or ego, it will cease to exist. Nothing could be further from the TRUTH.

Civilization, even on our planet, can be measured also in very great periods of time. Such civilizations are periodically dispersed or interrupted by geological phenomena — ice ages, floods, the changing of continents, shifting of the earth's axis, etc.— but the true picture of what actually takes place during such periods has been greatly distorted by geologists and archeologists who have drawn their conclusions from the limited data available to them. Consequently, our schools teach us of the ages of primeval creatures and how man eventually emerged in some sort of primitive form, gradually evolving into more and more of a "civilized" creature.

According to Yoga philosophy, man has been on this planet for many times the number of years generally accepted in western thought.

Furthermore, he was *never* a primitive creature; on the contrary, there have been "golden ages" during which he was an extremely civilized creature, perhaps far more so than he is today. (Naturally, you understand that in using the word "civilization," we are not talking about washing machines and refrigerators. We are referring to man's ability to perceive TRUTH and to apply such precepts to living in harmony with himself and his fellow man.)

We have stated that everything in this book would be practical; all information would pertain to everyday life and consist of techniques and knowledge which you could immediately apply. This must also be true of the Yoga philosophy and we therefore cannot dwell too long on Yoga cosmology. We must pass on and take up the practical aspect of "How the Yogi Sees the Universe" as it pertains to you and your everyday life.

We have briefly discussed the "day and night of creation." Now we shall find that *man himself has an individual day and night.* When his physical body has what we call "life," this is his "day." When his life expires, that is, his physical body dies, he passes into his "night." But just as the entire creation is eternal in its never-ending days and nights, so, the Yogi informs us, is the soul of man. The fact that the individual soul of man lives through many days and nights is what is known as *incarnation and reincarnation.*

Wherever we look, we see the forces of nature at work; not only the physical forces but the infinite subtle forces. It must be evident that there is a great intelligence inherent in all such forces. And because we know that such intelligence exists and that there is an incredible *order* in all things (however difficult such order is to perceive), we have been able to evolve "sciences" pertaining to many things.

Our sciences are founded primarily on the principle of cause and effect. We prove in the course of many experiments that if a certain thing is done in a certain manner, we can quite accurately predict the result or "effect"! Now does it not seem logical to you that the same intelligence, the same order, pervades the actions and thoughts of your everyday life? That is, would it not seem most probable that every action, every thought, everything which you *cause,* no matter how great or how slight, must, in some way, at some time, have an effect?

If you put your finger into a fire, you will get an immediate burn. This burn is an *immediate* effect; the fire is the cause. If you are careless regarding your health, if you dissipate and do not take care of your body, you will eventually fall ill from one disease or another. This illness is the result of many causes which preceded it. In this case the effect was delayed but nonetheless materialized. *You are continually generating causes.*

Everything that you do or say or think is a *cause* which must have an *effect* in some way, somewhere, at some time!

There is absolutely no exception to this law. Many of these effects are immediate as with the burn from the fire. But many of them are delayed, and if your physical body does not live long enough to have these effects work themselves out in it, this does not mean that these effects vanish. They remain in what we can call the "individual soul" during the night of one's existence. When the interval of the night is over, you are born again (reincarnated) in a physical body and in an environment which best provides the opportunity for the latent effects to manifest.

This helps to partially explain why people are born with what appears to be talent or genius in certain fields, "good" and "bad" luck, etc. These qualities are all the results of "effects" of their previous lives manifesting. The fact that an individual cannot understand why he was born with certain advantages or limitations, or that he feels he would do much better were he born in a different country or environment, is due again to the fact that the ordinary mind is unable to comprehend the divine wisdom, the perfect spiritual order of all things. *The sum total of effects which have to be worked out at any given moment in an individual's existence is known as his "karma."*

Now, not only are these effects continually working themselves out, but you are also continually creating *new* causes which in turn must work themselves out in varying periods of time. Therefore, it is truly spoken that "no thought or action is without its results." The fact that you may not be able to anticipate or forecast the result of any single action or series of actions does not mean that there will be no consequences of these actions. The Yogic approach to the question of karma goes far beyond morality, beyond "good" and "evil." In Yoga we do not attempt to learn and memorize a multitude of do's and don'ts, so that we know which ones to apply to a given situation. What happens is that one reacts correctly with deep intuition, not with thought, as he gradually becomes more and more aware of Universal Mind.

The crux of the whole matter of karma is this: If an individual is forever generating causes and if these causes must forever work out in effects, then this would seem to mean that an individual must be reborn eternally. "Exactly so," says the Yogi. This is what is depicted by the "eternal wheel of life"—the eternal births and deaths through which the individual soul must pass, always suffering and never finding the true peace which it seeks. Is there then no escape? Yes, there is, according to Yoga, one escape and only one escape.

Stop the Causes and There Are No Effects

But if every action is in itself a new cause,

how can the causes be stopped? The causes are stopped by *disassociation with your actions.* You act. You do what you have to do in your everyday life, but you act in such a way as not to be involved in your actions! In this way the action is not attached to you; there is consequently no cause and there can be no effect. You have withdrawn yourself from the entire matter. In other words, you are in the fire when necessary, but you are not being burned. You are engaged in living your life in the most complete manner possible and yet you are not being tossed about as a leaf in the wind. Does this seem difficult to understand and apply? Let us examine the matter more closely.

When you become upset, angry, jealous, anxious, overjoyed, depressed, etc., what is involved in these things? It is your mental and emotional bodies which create and experience such sensations. If the mental and emotional bodies were brought under control and not allowed to run away with you, as do the wild horses with the carriage when the driver of the coach falls asleep, then you would not be subject to cause and effect. The mental and emotional bodies are another way of speaking about the ego. You must expose the ego for what it is — *the illusion of a separate self.* We must be able first to control and then to see through the ego.

When you are able to do this, you will be free from the endless round of births and deaths. Only in this freedom can you experience the true peace which you are forever seeking. The droplet of water remains what it is only as long as it is detached from the ocean; when it joins the ocean it *becomes* the ocean and can no longer be distinguished as an individual droplet. The strangest of all ironies is that *you, too, have already joined the ocean of Universal Mind;* indeed, you could never have been separate from it for a moment, but the ego obscures this profound realization. To dissolve the ego so that it may merge with Universal Mind and your true identity be revealed to you is the purpose of the Yoga and primarily of the techniques of meditation.

Concentration with the Voice

We have previously used sight, sound and breath as our "passive" concentration techniques. Now we utilize the *voice!*

We have discussed the day and night of creation. The Yogi informs us that if we were able to hear the *sound* of the "day" as the creation was manifesting — indeed, if we could somehow stand outside of the universe and hear the *sum total* of all the sounds that were occurring in the universe, we would hear the great sound of OM. To become in harmony with the Universal Mind, the Yogi reproduces this sound with his voice in deep, long, steady tones. The effect of this sound is a most calming and, at the same time, energizing one. We are going to learn and use this technique.

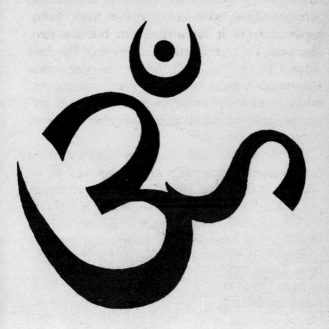

"*The Sanskrit symbol for OM,* the most powerful of all Yogic incantations (*Mantras*). Representing the entire range of creation, it is uttered (as instructed on the following page) to achieve unity with Universal Mind.

Seated in a cross-legged posture, keep your spine erect, form the circle *(mudra)* with your thumb and index finger of both hands and lower your eyelids as we have done in previous techniques. Slowly inhale a Complete Breath. Shape your lips in the form of an "O" and, keeping your voice as low and as steady as possible, use half of the air in your lungs to very slowly sound the letter "O." When half of the air has been used with this sound, close your lips and sound the letter "M," feeling the vibrations throughout your head and body. When you have used all of your air producing the "M" sound, without pause inhale another Complete Breath and repeat.

Perform this technique seven times. You must concentrate fully on the sounds all of the time they are being produced. Attempt to sink into the center of the sound. See if you can determine from whence it is originating. *Become the sound!* Keep your voice low and steady both in quality and pitch. Upon completion of the seven sounds, you will experience an indescribable calmness and elevation.

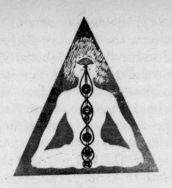

CHAPTER 7.

HOW THE YOGI
SEES
THE BODY

Let us briefly summarize the essence of the last chapter. The Yogic concept of the day and night of creation, of reincarnation and of karma, is of very great scope. The major premise is that man is subject to eternal births and deaths and consequently to never-ending suffering because he is imbued with the idea of a separate ego or self, and this self is involved in an infinite series of causes and effects in a vain effort to satisfy and fulfill itself.

The ultimate objective of the practice of Yoga (indeed, the very meaning of Yoga) is to merge this illusionary self with the ocean of Universal Mind so that cause and effect cease to be a reality and true peace is experienced.

To achieve this "liberation," we are engaging in the practices of both physical and mental Yoga. The meditation (and concentration) techniques are instrumental in effecting the gradual realization of Universal Mind, and for this purpose you are being presented with the classical Yogic techniques for "active" and "passive" meditation.

Now we shall attempt to make you aware that the practice of the Yoga physical exercises *(Hatha Yoga)* is of fundamental importance in achieving our objective.

The Yogi has, in certain vital areas, understood a great deal more concerning the functioning and purpose of the physical body and the mind than have the physiologists, biologists and psychologists of our age. The two major reasons why this fact is not better known are: (1) The true Yogi has never been interested in convincing the authorities of the Western World of the truth of his knowledge and realizations: he knows that it is impossible to present this knowledge within the extremely confining framework of what is known as "objective" and "analytical" science; (2) when he *has* expressed his knowledge, it has been in a symbolical and poetical manner, so that if the Yogic source books are read by the person not sufficiently versed in the Yogic style and symbols they appear to be incomprehensible.

However, when the "keys" are known, Yogic knowledge presents a much more complete and meaningful picture of the nature of body and mind than anything which is offered to us by the materialistic scientists of the West. (This statement is a generality many deep-thinking, more mystically inclined scientists and psychiatrists are more and more transcending the cold materialism of objective science and realizing the great truths inherent in eastern mysticism. The late C. Jung was one such person.)

The Yogi draws no distinction between what is supposedly "mystical" and therefore cannot be understood by the ordinary mind, and what is "objective" and "physical" and can therefore supposedly be grasped by this mind. The wise man knows that such distinctions are simply the workings of the ordinary mind (whose function, remember, is to create, observe and analyze such distinctions), and as such actually serve to confuse, not enlighten, one who seeks to "Know thyself."

Again, the *technical* aspects of what the Yogi knows about the structure and function of the physical and mental bodies is extremely complex, although by no means discouragingly so. While this information would undoubtedly be of very great interest to those persons involved in physiology and related sciences, we must assume that the person for whom this book is intended is much more concerned with the *practical application* of this Yogic knowledge to his own particular needs rather than its theoretical aspect.

That is why, at no time in any of my writings on Yoga, have I presented the reader with any material which I thought he could not apply almost immediately in one form or another. It has been my experience that as you expand consciousness through your Yoga and related studies, a great deal of technical knowledge is realized and grasped intuitively. The Yogi states that "as you realize Universal Mind you are in possession of all knowledge."

From the practical standpoint, therefore, here is a summary of the factors in the subject of "How the Yogi Sees the Body" as it pertains to *your* practice of Yoga.

There are great mental and physical forces within us which lie dormant; which are not being used. The practice of Yoga awakens these forces and as this occurs, the ordinary mind, our usual consciousness, is expanded. This expansion leads to increasing perception and awareness of the true nature of the universe, resulting in the eventual realization that man is SPIRIT or Universal Mind.

To the extent that this realization occurs, man merges with the ocean of Universal Consciousness and as such is "liberated" from the mundane or illusionary world of the ordinary mind and the ego. This experience which we have called "enlightenment" is also known by the important Sanskrit words *samadhi* and *nirvana*. The nature of such an experience is actually indescribable because, as it was already pointed out, the ordinary mind is not equipped to comprehend it. The questions which are always asked by the student in connection with the ultimate realization have to do with, "What will become of me when I *do* have this experience?"

But you must remember that it is the ordinary mind which is concerned with this question, because it believes that somehow or other it will cease to exist and the unknown is always a source of anxiety and insecurity. In reality it is *only* the merging of the self with the Universal Mind which can impart to you the peace and security you are seeking, and consequently you should make this the objective of the greater part of your life and not allow the infinite tricks and delusions of the ordinary mind to deter you from this goal.

Of course, there is also what we must call "faith" involved in this study. If you do not believe intuitively in the higher consciousness, in Universal Mind, it is pointless to proceed with the techniques, although I should like to state that I am aware of many, many people who began their study of Yoga strictly for the benefit which could be derived from the physical exercises and became deeply immersed in the philosophical pursuits as the exercises began to arouse dormant forces!

I should also like to clarify a point in connection with the realization of the higher consciousness. This realization is by no means *complete* and *permanent;* it may occur in varying time periods, from a few seconds to some hours and even days. Spiritual texts are replete with such examples of partial and temporary enlightenment. But once the student has caught a glimpse of the higher consciousness, he knows where the treasure lies and can never be permanently dissuaded from his quest after liberation, regardless of the interference, deterrents and great difficulties which he must often face in this quest.

Now let us see how and why the Yogi makes use of the great potential forces within the organism, in order to aid in the expansion of consciousness.

To begin with a simple illustration, picture an 8-cylinder engine which is functioning with 1 cylinder. The other 7 cylinders are not working. There is nothing wrong with the cylinders themselves, but the spark plugs upon which they are dependent are inactive. The inefficiency of an engine in this condition is obvious. But as the spark plugs were activated and each of the 7 cylinders was made to work in turn, not only would the strain be removed from the lone working cylinder, but the machine would become increasingly *efficient*. Now we can very well apply this illustration to our own organism (which, remember, is made up of our physical, mental and emotional bodies). The Yogi informs us that there are 7 major areas of tremendous *potential* force within this organism where great amounts of lifeforce are stored which could be used, but which are now dormant.

Because these areas lack the *spark* necessary to activate them, the stored life-force within them lies unused. Consequently, the organism, functioning with only a fraction of its potential power, is inefficient. This inefficiency manifests itself physically (the organism is easily subject to fatigue, discomfort, disease); mentally (the limitations of the ordinary mind); emotionally (continual enslavement to fear, anxiety, insecurity, depression, as well as the intense desire and attachment to their opposites, security, happiness, etc.)

Six of these areas of potential force have their focal point or control board at six ascending points along a microscopic avenue situated in the middle of the spinal column. These focal points are called *centers (chakras)*. The spark which is necessary to activate or "open" these centers and release the forces which they control lies at the base of this microscopic cord and is known by the Sanskrit word *kundalini*. This word may be translated as *basic power*.

When stimulated and aroused, the basic power makes an ascending journey up through the cord within the spinal column and according to how far it is made to rise, activates and opens, partially or fully, the various centers. These centers then begin to "work;" the areas of force in different parts of the organism over which they have control are also awakened and their great storehouse of life-force is made available. This increased life force working within the organism helps to produce the expansion of consciousness.

It is through the gradual awakening and control of the centers that Yogis derive what is often referred to as "super-natural powers" and "extra-sensory perception." These powers are looked upon by true Yogis only as an indication that a certain stage in their study has been reached. They are not an end, but simply a sign along the path. If and when such powers are actually utilized by the Yogi, it is under extraordinary circumstances and only for service to his fellow beings.

If powers are employed in any harmful or destructive manner or for self-enrichment, they are the undoing of the one who so utilizes them. There is a severe warning regarding this fact which is given by the guru to the student. To idly exhibit any power which has been gained through Yoga practice is to greatly circumscribe one's progress. The exhibitionists in the Orient who perform feats of self-hypnosis for favors are known as *fakirs* and are not to be confused with Yogis.

The basic power, as it is activated and makes its ascending journey, generally opens up only one center at a time. The lowest centers are the first to be opened (those which correspond to the reproductive system and the organs and glands of the viscera), then the middle centers (those of the solar plexus

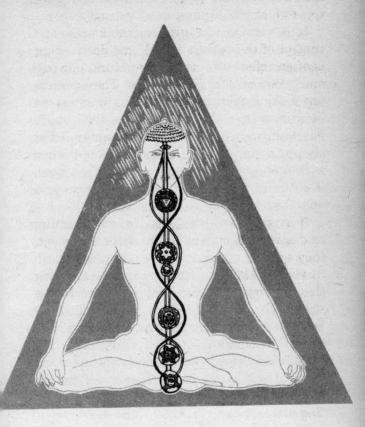

The 7 centers of force which are opened through the journey of the Basic Power.

and the heart), and finally the highest centers (the throat or thyroid gland, the pineal gland, or "third eye)."

There are detailed descriptions as well as names and symbols regarding each of the centers; it is not of practical value to discuss the specific powers and values of the separate centers in this text. The interested reader is referred to *The Serpent Power*, by Arthur Avalon, Ganesh and Company, India, if authentic, detailed information is desired.

The seventh center, known as the "thousand petal lotus," corresponds not only to the physical brain but actually extends beyond the skull. See the broken lines surrounding the head in the illustration of the seven centers of force.

The basic power will not be awakened until the organism has been purified and made sufficiently strong to receive and conduct the greater forces which are released in this journey. This purification and strengthening process is the major objective of physical *(hatha)* Yoga and each of the techniques of meditation aids the process. It is most interesting for the student to note that the "health" aspects of the physical exercises are actually a by-product of Hatha Yoga. Its basic purpose is purification and strengthening of the organism followed by the gradual stimulation of the centers.

The basic power must never, under any circumstances, be *forced* to rise. That is why you must always carefully follow the directions given to you in the Exercise Books for performing the physical postures and never strain. If you proceed with moderation, patience and self-control, you will gain the health and strength of the nervous system before the possibility of awakening the basic power has to be considered.

Directing the Life-Force

In Chapter 5 we discussed the life-force in detail. It was stated that the life-force could be controlled and directed with very positive results. It is possible to consciously direct the life-force from one point in the organism where it has been stored to another point for purposes of alleviating pain, illness and other negative conditions. This is also a wonderful technique to use for a quick recharging.

In addition, the life-force can be directed into the body of another person to promote healing. That which is called "magnetic healing" is performed either consciously or subconsciously by people who are able to accumulate extra life-force and then transfer it to the point where it is needed.

One of the major centers for the storage of life-force is the *solar plexus* (sun center), which is located in the pit of the abdomen and which is a vast network of nerves. Let us assume that the supply of life-force is to be sent into the *head* for relieving a headache, or simply for general relaxation and relief of tension. (We could choose any other area of the organism.) Assume a comfortable sitting or lying posture. If sitting, use a cross-legged position. Place the fingertips of both hands lightly on your solar plexus (that very sensitive spot at the top of the abdomen beneath the ribs). Keep your fingers lightly on the solar plexus and slowly inhale a Complete Breath.

As you inhale, forcefully direct the life-force into the solar plexus by drawing it through your nostrils and lungs, and finally direct it into your fingertips. In your mind, form an image of pure energy, like the flowing of an intense white light which floods your entire body as you inhale and which is drawn into your fingertips. You must concentrate very intensely upon holding the image of this white light in your mind (Figure 11).

When you have completed the inhalation, place the fingertips of both hands on your forehead between your eyebrows. Hold your breath for the several seconds required to slowly transfer the fingers from the solar plexus to the head. Now exhale very slowly and, as you do so, picture the white light flowing from your fingertips into your head,

FIG. 11 *The fingers are placed on the solar plexus and the white light is pictured flowing into them.*

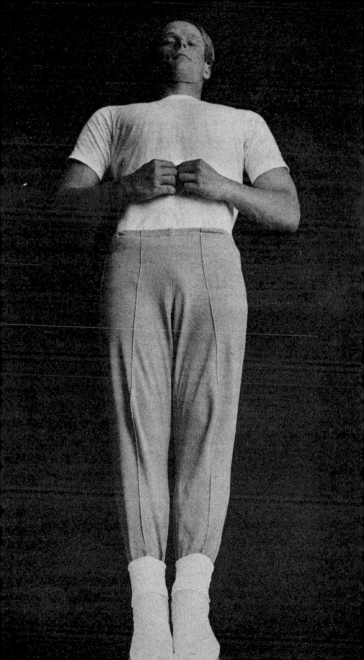

completely flooding the head with the life-force.

You will gradually begin to feel a pleasant tingling throughout the area into which the life-force is being directed and it will slowly grow warm (Figure 12). When your breath has been completely exhaled, slowly return your fingers to the solar plexus and repeat the process. Try always, during this entire procedure, to retain the image of the white light in your mind's eye. The white light is the point of concentration for this technique.

For best results you should perform this technique from 7 to 21 times according to the time available to you and the serious-ness of the disturbance. It usually requires approximately 14 repetitions in the beginning before you can expect to experience any re-sults. If the disturbance is a serious one, rest for several minutes after performing the 21 repetitions and then continue to re-peat in groups of 21.

Remember that you can direct the life-force to any area of the body. If your shoulder required attention, you would transfer the fingertips from the solar plexus to the should-er, etc. This is a fundamental practice in Yoga to raise the vibrations of an afflicted area of

FIG. 12   *The fingers are transferred to the "third eye" area and the white light is pic-tured flooding the head.*

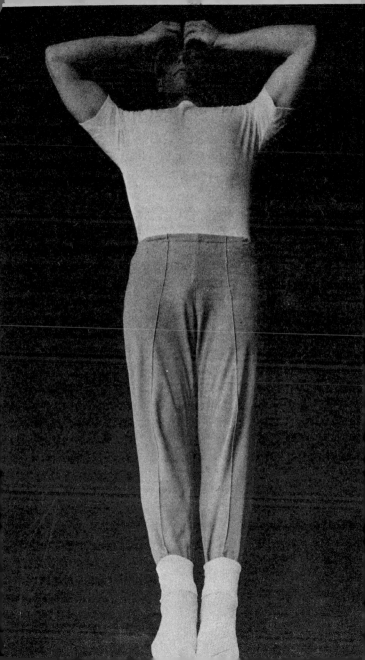

the organism and to help restore it to normal functioning. It is used specifically: as a strong refresher and revitalizer of the mind and body; a quick recharge for the storage battery of the organism; to relieve pain and discomforts; to promote relaxation, especially from emotional and nervous tension. It has also proved to be an excellent method for overcoming insomnia.

If the reclining posture or the cross-legged position is impractical, or interferes with directing the life-force into the disturbed region, then perform this technique in any convenient comfortable position. The important point is to have both the solar plexus and the area into which the life-force must flow accessible to the fingertips.

If no visible relief or improvement is immediately apparent, do not be discouraged, but continue the practice as advised. Remember, the force with which you are working is very *real*, although *subtle*. It often requires a period of time to gain ability with this technique, but how well worth the effort!

After you have gained some mastery in directing the life-force, you can apply the technique to aid others. In this case, the first part of the technique remains the same, i.e., your inhalation of the Complete Breath with your fingers on your solar plexus. But in the transference, the fingertips are placed on the afflicted area of the other person's body and you direct the flow of the white light and life-force into this area during the exhalation. The person with whom you are working should attempt to cooperate in seeing the white light if possible. If they are not able to cooperate for one reason or another, you may still proceed without their help. However, do not attempt to work with anyone who scoffs at the idea or who does not want this type of help.

When you have gained real mastery of the technique, you will find that you are able to direct and transmit the life-force with thought alone and no physical contact with the solar plexus will be necessary!

मणिपद्मेहूँ

"OM MA-NI PAD-ME HŪṂ"

CHAPTER 8.

WHO ARE YOU?

In the very first sentence of this book, we inquired, "Who are you?" We must now look more deeply into this very profound question and determine how it can be of use to us. We have frequently used the words "you" and "your" in these pages. We have said such things as "Is it really *you*?" "*You* observe *your* body and mind," "*You* have imprisoned yourself," etc. Now we must ask in all seriousness, "Who is this *you* that we are speaking about?" Indeed, let us repeat the original question, "Who are you?"

You might quickly answer this peculiar question with your name: "John Brown" or "Mary Smith." "But," the Yogi would reply, "that is just the name which has been given to you. Who are YOU?"

And so you might have to search a little farther to explain who you were. You might tell your address, family, friends, clubs and organizations to which you belong, social activities, religious and philosophical beliefs, and so forth. But you would always be telling something *about* yourself, trying to explain yourself in relation to the other people and other conditions in your life. You would then begin to see, if you were questioned long enough, that the "you" or the "I" about which we are continually speaking, *has no separate existence but lives only in relation to other things, other people!* You would eventually discover, probably much to your astonishment, that you are really not at all who you *think* you are, or whom other people and eternal circumstances have led you to believe you are! The more you attempted to explain yourself under the above kind of questioning, the more difficult it would become to do so.

We have what we believe is an *identity*. Just as we carry some form of identification — driver's license, credit cards, etc. — to prove who we are when it is necessary to do so, so does your ordinary mind carry its own identity card to prove that this "you" is quite real. But just as the identity card in your pocket is not really you but merely certain statistics *about* you, so it is that the identity card that your mind carries and speaks about with such assurance and certainty is only a group of compiled statistics and not really YOU.

This "I" which we are continually referring to owes its existence to the ordinary mind, which has created or manufactured it, and keeps it alive through a most deceiving process. The fact that this "I" is referred to in authoritative philosophical literature as the "ego" seems to lend a certain validity and reality to something which you will find is really as elusive as a shadow when you try to take hold of it.

"Well," you may say, "I might have difficulty explaining to someone else who I am, but *I* certainly know who I am." In this case the Yogi would press you still farther with his questioning. "*Who* is it that knows who you are? Are there two yous: one who is there and the other who knows he is there? And *who* is the you that can think that there are two yous? In that case, there must be *three* yous: (1) the original you; (2) the you that is thinking about you; (3) the you that is thinking about the you that is thinking about you."

Once we start this chain, it extends into infinity, like placing two mirrors face to face and trying to figure out which mirror is reflecting how many images of itself and how many images of the other mirror. Which is the *real you*? You may answer, "The first one." But how can this first you really be you when he exists only if there is *another you* to think about him? And how can the second you be the real one if it takes a third to realize the second you is thinking about the first one?

Read these above paragraphs over again slowly if they seem confusing, and you will understand how it is that by the very logic which the ordinary mind so extols, we can prove that the YOU which is being carried about is a phantom and actually has no *real* existence. This *you* appears to be the real person only when you reach into the file that the ordinary mind has labelled: "You" (or "I").

We must have the realization that this ordinary mind-machine processes data and selects for us "likes" and "dislikes," "beliefs" and "disbeliefs," gradually building a giant file of facts which it labels "I." And it does its very best to say, "I believe," "I think," "I like," etc. Thus the I is nourished and inflated. Now in order to truly realize how the ordinary mind (which in this work is considered as synonomous with the ego and the I) keeps you in perpetual pursuit without ever bringing you any closer to true peace, security, fulfillment and liberation from endless suffering, desire, fear and anxiety, you must transcend the ordinary mind and grasp this idea of the illusionary "I" with the Universal Mind. But of course the difficulty involved in accomplishing this is that the ordinary mind cannot conceive of such a thing as "transcending" itself! In short, you cannot debate or reason your way beyond your ordinary mind; this is like trying to pull yourself up by your own bootstraps.

If you would transcend the ordinary mind and see the universe and the true nature of your "self," you must allow your ordinary mind to *dissolve* into the Universal Mind. This begins to occur as you practice the various techniques of physical and mental Yoga. It is most important for the student to be clear regarding this point: It should not be thought that there are really two minds — an ordinary mind and a Universal Mind. There is only one MIND. But because we have come to rely so strongly upon our ordinary mind and its machinations, its logic, reason and ability to debate, analyze and compute with so-called "objectivity," we are unable to see it as only an aspect of the Universal Mind.

"But," the student asks, "how can you eliminate reason and logic? And what will happen to me if I should succeed in doing so?" Here again, the difficulty involved is in not being able to perceive that it is only the ordinary mind that is concerned with its own phantom. There is no real "fear" apart from the ordinary mind. *The concept of fear and the ordinary mind are one and the same thing!* The ordinary mind creates these ideas and then appears to deal with them. The mind endlessly creates problems (which, remember, is part of its function) and then gives the impression of solving these problems. But it is simultaneously creating additional problems. One is thus led to believe that the problems are external, on the outside, and the solution to the problems comes from within, from his mind. He does not perceive that *the problem and the solution arise from the same source!*

Let us examine from a slightly different vantage point how one may realize the Universal Mind, joining his tiny particle of ego consciousness with the ocean of Universal Consciousness.

Imagine a circle with a point in the exact center. Let the *circumference* of this circle represent the ordinary mind, and the *center* of the circle represent the Universal Mind. Remember, however, that only the ordinary mind thinks in terms of "circumferences" and "centers." It is only the ordinary mind that is confined to the world of reason and logic. The Universal Mind is always at the center of everything — so much so that even the idea of a "center" has no absolute reality.

As we attempt to present an insight into Universal Mind with this imagery, we must alternate between the circumference and center of the circle. When we are on the circumference, our terms will be logical, rational, reasonable, all of which the ordinary mind can understand. But when we wish to have you tra scend or escape the confines of your ordinary mind, we must "jump" into the center of the circle, where our concepts and the words we use may be incoherent or confusing to the ordinary mind.

We alternate in this manner because if we do so often enough, the reader may at some point jump into the center without even being aware that he is doing so. When this occurs, even for a few moments, everything concerning the nature of the Universal Mind will at once be clear and no further explanation will be necessary. In the study of Zen Buddhism, this type of realization is known as "sudden enlightenment."

The ordinary mind is, therefore, to be pictured as the circumference of a circle. Our cherished reason and logic will continually move us from one part of the circumference to another (giving us the illusion of movement; movement to the ordinary mind is associated with "progress"), but actually never any closer to the *center*. Reason can never reason itself away or logic transport us beyond logic, however intricate or seemingly profound they become.

The ordinary mind sustains itself in terms of opposites, continually alternating between one extreme and the other. That is how it reasons and makes decisions. It determines how good something is by measuring it against varying degrees of bad; it presents a picture of joy by contrasting it with despair. It will have you believe that not only is there an *I* (which it perpetuates as we have discussed), but that there is a *good I* and a *bad I* — and that through your ingenuity and resourcefulness the good *I* will engage in battle with the bad *I* and overcome him.

And around and around the circumference of the circle you go, the good *I* in a desperate chase to catch up with the bad *I* so that he can fix up the bad *I* and make him as good as the good *I*. Do you see what an impossible task the ordinary mind has undertaken for you? The good *I* can no more catch up with the bad *I* and reform him than one end of a stick can catch up with the opposite end. The good *I* in all of his goodness and the bad *I* in all of his badness spring from the same source and both are phantoms, shadows manufactured by the ordinary mind, having no real existence. You may like to think of the real you as being associated with the good *I* in alliance against the bad *I,* but if so, you again have at least *three yous:* (1) an original *I* who is allied with the (2) good *I* who are in battle to subdue the (3) bad *I.* In the midst of all this confusion, where are YOU?

At this point, you may assert: "But I *know* that I have bad habits, bad traits, bad qualities. Shouldn't I try to rid myself of these negative things?" "Of course you should," answers the Yogi, "but you must understand what you are doing, otherwise your efforts are completely misdirected." He implies that since you do not understand the nature of the *I* to begin with; since you do not know from where he came, or where he is now, or if he is real at all; since you know next to nothing of this shadow called the *I*, how can you make use of him to fix himself up?

The serious error which is being made by so many people, especially in our age of psychology, psychiatry and self-improvement, lies in the attempt to investigate the *I*, the ordinary mind, so that they may analyze its nature and how to cope with it. But this type of investigation is what the Yogi would mean by "misdirected effort," because what takes place is that the ordinary mind is being investigated by the ordinary mind. This is like the dog trying to catch his own tail. *The ordinary mind can never determine the nature of the ordinary mind.*

Thus we may conclude that everything which strengthens the illusion of the *I* prevents us from functioning at the center of the circle where the self is transcended and where our true peace and security lie. But here again, one must always be aware that the ordinary mind cannot truly conceive of the nature of *real peace and security,* because the ordinary mind thinks of such things only in relation to their opposites, in this instance, *restlessness and insecurity.* That is why ordinary mind can never know Universal Mind; because when it hears these words it thinks of *something.*

Even if it thinks that these ideas are too great for it to understand, it is still *thinking*. In other words, all concepts which the ordinary mind may have concerning peace, liberation, or the center of the circle are merely thoughts and images and as such cannot represent the true nature, the *reality* of such things.

Do not think for a moment that by transcending the *I* or merging the self, you are giving up something. Nothing is lost. But we must make use of the words "lost" or "give up" to prepare the ordinary mind to take its "jump." Remember that only the ordinary mind is concerned about losing itself (as though such a thing could actually occur). The fact is, that since there is no reality to the *I* (and you will come gradually to realize this truth), there is nothing to lose. We speak about a "jump" because only from the circumference of the circle does it appear that something will change or be lost. From the center, you truly understand that nothing can change and that there is no center about which to speak.

But such an idea can only be understood from the vantage point other than the one which the ordinary mind maintains. The point at which we are aiming is the point which is not really a point! All of the paradoxes in these pages — speaking about going somewhere when there is nowhere to go; telling *you* to understand something when there is *no you* to understand it; advising you to give up something when there is actually nothing to give up — are merely continual alternations between the circumference and the center in the hope, as previously pointed out, that you may suddenly jump beyond your ordinary mind, in which case you will instantaneously comprehend the nature of Universal Mind.

In that state of Universal Mind to which we have been referring as the "center of the circle," one knows the nature of his own being and becomes *whole*. He remains in this state only as long as he has no knowledge of an individual self or *I*. Once the *I* takes over and one says to himself, "Now I am in the center of the circle," he is at once back on the circumference. Having no self and no ordinary mind automatically places one in the center. Knowledge of a self and a mind must put one on the circumference.

The ego now rears his head and says, "But I don't want to lose my individuality." Again we must explain that only the ego thinks that something is lost, because only the ego is concerned about loss or gain. What the ego is thinking of as "individuality" and of the ability to think in logical, rational terms is in reality the very prison from which we want to escape.

In reproductions and replicas of many sages, saints, Buddhas and enlightened men of the east, you will notice that there seems to be a subtle smile playing around the lips.

We are told that this is because, when these persons attained to the state of enlightenment, they could not help but smile as they realized man's folly in imprisoning himself within the confines of the ego. How simple it is to be free and how difficult man has made it for himself to gain this freedom!

All of the great spiritual leaders have spoken and acted from the center of the circle. This is what often makes their words and actions difficult for the ordinary mind to comprehend. The prophets of the Old Testament, Jesus, Buddha, Lao-Tzu, explained and taught in their individual styles the things that are required for a man to live and act in the center. All great works of art, whether sculpture, painting, music or literature, are conceived and executed from the center. That is why such works have about them the permanence of *truth* which renders them great and alive throughout all the ages.

At the center there can be no wrong. The arbitrary concept of the ordinary mind concerning right and wrong, good and evil, ceases to exist. It is swallowed up in the truth of the Universal Mind. All movements, thoughts, words emanating from the center are attributes of truth. In the center, one is free, and although the fire is burning all about him, the center is not touched.

In the very midst of everyday life one may exist in the center. One can engage in all of the actions that seem to contribute to the confusion of everyday living and yet be apart from them. This has nothing to do with using your "will power" to make yourself calm or disinterested; that would be only another device of the ordinary mind. There is no self-hypnosis or deluding one's self in the practice of Yoga. On the contrary, it is the one study which permits no deception whatsoever and in which the student is methodically led to the ultimate confrontation of the self.

One of the greatest Yogis of the century — Ramana Maharshi of India — advocated a very basic meditation technique for investigating the self, the I. The student, seating himself in the cross-legged posture, proceeds to ask silently, "Who am I?" He then waits to hear the answer provided by the ordinary mind. The object is not to analyze the answers in an attempt to determine their merit, but rather to learn all of the statistics that the ordinary mind has stored away under the label of I.

As you continue to ask yourself, "Who am I?" for several minutes each time you work with this technique, you gradually come to realize that all of the facts and figures of the ordinary mind regarding the entity which it has built into the I *are only statistics* and that none of these statistics are able to touch the heart of the matter. They cannot provide you with a true answer to this strange question.

This is not an intellectual problem, a puzzle or a riddle to be solved through ingenuity.

This is a technique which attempts to elicit an *experience*. As you continue to ask the questions, the ordinary mind itself begins to realize its inability to provide a true answer. This realization is of paramount importance, but the process cannot be accelerated through intellectual reasoning; it takes place during the patient practice of the exercise. The ordinary mind, being very clever and tricky, will attempt to convince you in every possible way of the uselessness and waste of time in asking this question. But if you persevere, you will find this to be one of the most revealing methods with which to expose the false and illusionary nature of what we call our self and of pointing the way to the center of the circle.

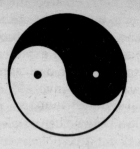

CHAPTER 9.

THE ART
OF
EXPERIENCING

The process of *naming* things and referring to them with words often leads us to *mistake the name and form of an object for the object itself.* We believe that when we have named an object, emotion or experience, we then *know and understand it.* Actually, the name or "label" which we use serves as a substitute for *experience* and our lives assume more and more the mechanical quality of the ordinary mind. We speak and think in words alone, taking for granted that we understand what is represented by them. Before very long the symbol reigns supreme, experience becomes less and less frequent and we find ourselves faced with apparently insurmountable problems which have actually been created for us by these symbols. The inability of the ordinary mind to *experience,* and the manner in which it prevents the entire organism from experiencing, is the primary reason for these problems.

To illustrate what is involved, let us utilize mathematical symbols, numbers. Numbers are a convenience. Take the number "5". You accept a check for five dollars if you believe that the check is "good." It *is* good if the required number of dollars are in the bank. The check is not the *real* five dollars; it is a convenient substitute. The symbol "5" has no value of its own. It has value only if what it supposedly represents really exists. Because most checks *do* have the necessary backing, we are able to conduct a vast number of transactions through checks. Millions of checks change hands in the faith that dollars are actually there to back them up, and that the gold and silver reserves are behind the dollars. This analogy may be applied to our own lives which are permeated with this interchange of symbols, often with tragic consequences. We are forever talking *about* living, *about* experiencing, but are the living and experiencing really there to back up the convenience of the symbols, the words?

At this point we arrive once more at the image of the center and the circumference of the circle. The center of the circle here becomes "experience and life" and the circumference is "thought and thinking about experiencing." Either you are *naming, thinking and speaking* about something and thus existing on the circumference, or you are *experiencing,* in which case you are in the center. What has happened to us is that the ordinary mind — the machine — spends most of its time presenting images *about* something, *but it is never able to experience anything!*

We have already seen that the ordinary mind is always telling you something about yourself in relation to other things but it is unable to tell you who you really are. It cannot *experience;* it can only *think* about experiencing. The more time you spend thinking about what you are going to do; how you are going to spend your money; how you will enjoy your leisure time; how you expect things to turn out next year, the less you are going to be living and experiencing *now.* Once you begin to chase the phantoms you will forever think *about* what you are going to experience, not what you are *now experiencing.* As such, you are only *thinking* about life, about reality, about the center, never really *living.*

Two violinists perform the same concerto. One has the ability to transcend the *I;* he has lost his self within the music. He does not play the music; the music is playing, flowing through *him.* His recital has the element of pure truth about it because the music springs spontaneously from the center. It is perfect and this perfection is projected into the core of his listeners. The second violinist possesses the same technical skill as the first. He plays the same music with the same orchestra. But he retains the concept that it is *he* performing the concerto. He has not been able to transcend the *I;* consequently he is not playing from the center. His performance may be perfect technically but it is not *alive.* He does not transmit *experience* to his audience.

So, too, are we not alive on the circumference. We are never at the heart of the matter; we do not exist as embodiments of truth. We are always speaking or thinking *about* a thing, always chasing the shadow, continually grasping for something which is forever just beyond our reach, hoping and conspiring for the phantom of a future happiness, unable to *experience* the truth of the present moment, of the NOW!

The function of the symphonic conductor is to make the entire orchestra experience — *become* — the music, not simply perform it. Nothing is actually given up or lost by the individual in these cases. Indeed, it is only when the *I* is dissolved that "style" and "personality" become genuine according to the true nature of the performer or the group, and are not simply technique and imitation. For the artist in any field to create a style which is individual and original, he must execute his art from the center; he must experience; he must transcend the self. In the writings of all great religions and all great philosophies we read that "in order to *find* yourself, you must learn to *lose* yourself."

Hence it would seem that the answer to that classical question, "Who am I?" would be, *"I am what I experience, no more, no less!"* Notice, not "what I experienc*ed*" (past), or "what I *will* experience" (future), but *"what I am now experiencing!"* Remember that we have already shown past and future experience to be a trick of the ordinary mind, abstractions which it can only think about *now*. So we must ask you, "Are you experiencing, or are you spending most of your time thinking about what you experienced or what you will experience?" If you work with the technique "Who am I?" as outlined in the previous chapter, you may discover that the greater part of each day, and indeed, the greater part of your entire life, is spent in *thinking about living, not in living itself!*

It is the understanding of *how to experience* that holds the solution to many of the terrible problems which confront us and involve the dreaded dragons of fear, anxiety, pain, insecurity and loss. But can you see that here again it is the ordinary mind which is writing the checks of "fear," "insecurity," etc., and we have come to rely upon the irrefutable authority of this ordinary mind to such a degree that we no longer question whether the "fear" and "insecurity" are actually in the bank. If you take a closer look, you will discover that it is the *thought* of pain, insecurity, loss which keeps you in bondage, because we are always attempting to *escape* these things. Consequently, the thoughts regarding them are forever with us. But the faster you try to run away; the more secure you seek to make your position; the more you resist loss; the more you attempt to avoid pain, the harder they breathe down your neck and the more impossible they become to leave behind.

You must realize, according to the Yoga philosophy, that there is no *real, objective fear, insecurity or loss*. There is only the ordinary mind's image of certain vague conditions which it has labeled "suffering," "fear," etc. It has convinced you that these must be avoided because they are a threat to the self. Thus these worrisome images sap your life-force since they make you devote most of your efforts to escaping them, to escaping the very things which the ordinary mind itself is manufacturing! How can ordinary mind escape ordinary mind? Impossible! But nonetheless, ordinary mind would have you protect the self regardless of what this entails (and it entails all of the absurd activities which the ordinary mind tells you must be undertaken).

We all know what it is like to be worried and anxious about something which we fear is going to happen to us. We can spend days, weeks and even years in dreadful anticipation of the situation which we fear is going to materialize. As time wears on we become exhausted by the anxiety. Eventually, from sheer weariness, we are forced to give in to the fear and we exclaim to ourselves, "I don't care anymore. I'm tired of worrying; I give up. Let the worst happen!"

The very moment that you sincerely make this decision, not only are you freed from the fear, but you find that even if the dreaded situation *should* materialize (which it most often does not), it cannot be one fraction of what you anticipated. You have surrendered yourself to *experience* and the actual experience can never be what the ordinary mind has imagined. You will free yourself from the image of fear and from all such images through your willingness to *feel* and *experience,* through your acceptance of whatever the experience may be. Thus our "fear" is a label of the ordinary mind, a label conjuring up frightful images which are the *symbols of the experience, but never the experience itself!*

To experience then, is to *become the thing* which is to be experienced. As we have already seen, there is no "self" who experiences. There is only pure, spotless experience. The ancient Yoga techniques of meditation teach us how to *become* the thing on which we are concentrating. There cannot be an object and one who sees the object. That which sees and that which is seen are one!

Experience as a Form of Meditation

Let us now turn, once again, to an *active* method of meditation, using *experience* as the basis.

As you engage in each of your activities throughout the day, *do not resist any experience.* Attempt to be aware of the essence of everything you are doing. Even in those everyday chores that you usually accomplish in a mechanical manner and which seem to be very boring, attempt to experience the nature of what you are doing. When you find yourself in what you have usually thought of as an "unpleasant" situation, do not resist it. Throw yourself into the center of the situation. Feel it; experience it. Remember that pain is not *painful* — it is something else, something far different from what the ordinary mind would have you believe.

The same is true with the everyday occurrences which we attempt desperately to avoid because we are trying to protect the self from unpleasant experiences. What the ordinary mind has labeled "unpleasant" will not be unpleasant if you will but decide to experience and not resist. The ordinary mind has convinced you of the nature of unpleasantness, but this is only its image, not the reality of experience. The moment you stop holding off what you consider to be a "negative" thing, you have automatically released yourself from the anxiety which this thing supposedly represents. You have also released vast amounts of life-force which are tied up in our multitude of resistances.

Ceasing to resist does not imply being irresponsible or disinterested. Rather, it means that you will always willingly face the dragons as they appear and never allow the "labels" of the ordinary mind to prevent you from *experiencing and knowing*. But you cannot "trick" yourself into experience to see whether or not it will "work." Every moment of your life must become genuine experience. When, without hesitancy or reservation, you become one with the stream of life, you experience each moment as it truly is, no longer vulnerable to the continual suffering and anxieties which can make everyday living fraught with apprehension.

Whenever you perceive that your life is assuming a mechanical nature, you must become aware of the fact that you have ceased to experience. Then use the various techniques which we have learned to merge yourself once again with the stream of life. *Jump into the center and experience!*

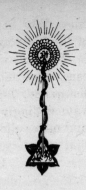

CHAPTER 10.

MEDITATION
WITHOUT SEED:
A SUMMARY

The ultimate achievement in the practice of Yoga is the continual experience of genuine peace and joy. This state is known as "pure bliss consciousness" and lies, as we have discussed, beyond the ordinary mind and the manner in which it interprets the everyday world. Therefore, the ordinary mind must be transcended. This is accomplished in Yoga through the practice of meditation. Meditation is not intellectual understanding; it is an *experience*.

Meditation is of two kinds, *active* and *passive*. The elementary active techniques which we learned in the early chapters of this manual take the form of observation of body and ordinary mind in action. As such, they can be applied at anytime and anywhere in everyday life. The advanced active meditation technique, learned in the previous chapter, cultivates the ability to continually experience and to do away with the desire of the ordinary mind to resist experience.

The passive techniques are reserved for practice in quiet and privacy. When proper conditions prevail, you may practice any of the passive techniques already learned. These were all meditation "with seed;" that is, you were given something upon which to meditate, a candle, the sound of OM, the lifeforce, the breath and so forth. Now, advanced passive meditation, known as "meditation without seed," will take *no form whatsoever*.

If you conscientiously practice the previous meditation techniques until you gain some mastery of them, you will be ready to attempt "meditation without seed." In the beginning, this type of meditation must be practiced in a completely quiet environment. Sit in one of the Lotus postures. Let the forefinger touch the thumb and lower the eyelids as already described. During this practice, all thoughts and perceptions of the ordinary mind are discarded. All thoughts and perceptions which arise are cast gently but firmly aside. In other words, you *stop thinking*. The moment you realize you *are* thinking, simply *will* the thoughts away. Practice this technique for approximately three minutes. You must continually be aware of arising thoughts or you will lose many seconds in distraction.

Through this technique you are gradually able to "shut off" the ordinary mind for several minutes each day and you will soon become aware of the inestimable value of being able to do so. Gradually you will be able to make "meditation without seed" an *active* technique and practice it for purposes of relaxation whenever you have a few spare moments during the day. It thus becomes possible to shut off the machine-like ordinary mind whenever you wish to do so. When the ordinary mind is quiet then you are truly *experiencing;* you revert to your natural state which is that of Universal Mind. When thoughts and perceptions are not permitted to arise, the mind does not become "blank;" it *expands!* Through this expansion, the ordinary mind is more and more in contact with Universal Mind.

No amount of thought, reason, debate, analysis or logic will provide the peace and liberation of body and mind which you are seeking. But the proper practice of your Yoga physical and meditation techniques will impart freedom and serenity. The directions for correct execution of both the physical and meditation exercises are presented in this text.

Practice regularly each day but *never become attached to your labors or look eagerly for results.* The fruits of your labor manifest more readily if you are not eagerly anticipating them.

Gradually, your entire life will become a strong, positive, quiet form of meditation. As you gain ability to control your ordinary mind through meditation, you will find that your life changes accordingly. Situations and conditions lose their power to disturb you, to make you restless, to cause suffering and confusion. It is not a question of "solving" problems; it becomes a matter of problems ceasing to arise (because the ordinary mind which manufactures the problems becomes less active, less frantic).

All of the states of mind and spirit that you have heard of in connection with "truth," "love," "brotherhood," "spirit," "God" are realized through meditation. If you are serious about the study of Yoga (or related studies), you will meditate as often as possible, utilizing one or more of the techniques you have learned. You will allow nothing to deter you from these practices. Each moment that you put into any form of meditation produces results beyond the imagination!

SECTION II

THE
POSTURE
ROUTINE
(Asanas)

THE
POSTURE
ROUTINE

In this section you will find a suggested routine of Yoga exercises *(asanas)* which will serve as preparation for meditation. This is not to be considered as a complete program of the postures, but only as a selection of techniques which will, in a brief period of time, impart the vitality and tranquility necessary to meditate to the greatest advantage.

The exercises in the following routine should be performed in the exact order of presentation. If you are already familiar with these postures from my other writings, the routine will present no problem. If you will be performing the postures for the first time, you must pay careful attention to the directions so that you learn and practice correctly.

As you become adept in the routine you should not pause between the exercises (unless instructed to do so in the directions) but rather perform them in a continuous manner, making the movements of one posture *flow*, like a dance, into the next. The entire routine, once learned, should require approximately fifteen minutes to complete, and this should be followed directly with a period of meditation approximately ten to twenty minutes in duration:

The following important points pertain to your practice:

1. For practice, choose a quiet place with a good supply of fresh air.
2. Remove all tight and confining clothing, including belt, watch, shoes and glasses. Actually, the less clothing, the better.
3. Use the same mat or pad for your practice every day. Do not allow it to be used for any other purpose.
4. Do not practice for at least ninety minutes after eating. You may eat after practicing if you wish.

Let us repeat: The following routine of *asanas* is offered only as a preparation for meditation. A complete routine of Yoga postures as a means of physical fitness and therapy is presented in the author's Yoga record albums and exercise books.

COMPLETE BREATH STANDING
(Figs. 1-5)

FIG. 1 *Stand as illustrated. Exhale deeply.*

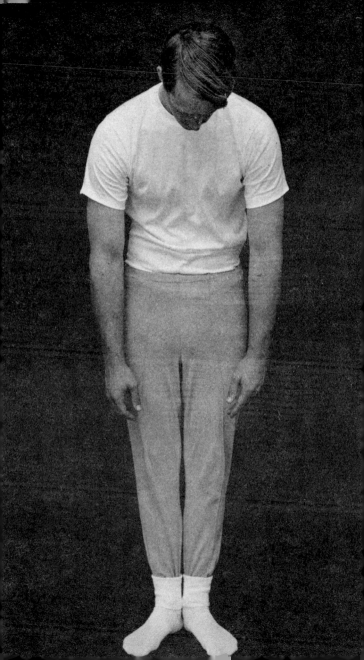

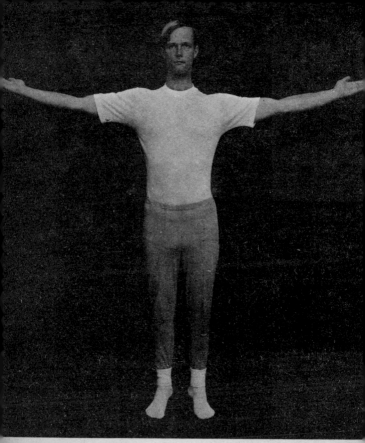

FIG. 2 *Slowly raise the arms as illustrated and begin to come up on toes. Simultaneously inhale and perform the abdominal and chest movements of the Complete Breath as you have learned in Section I.*

FIG. 3 *Continue the inhalation; also continue the raising of the arms until the hands touch overhead. Stand on the tips of your toes. The deep inhalation is now completed.*

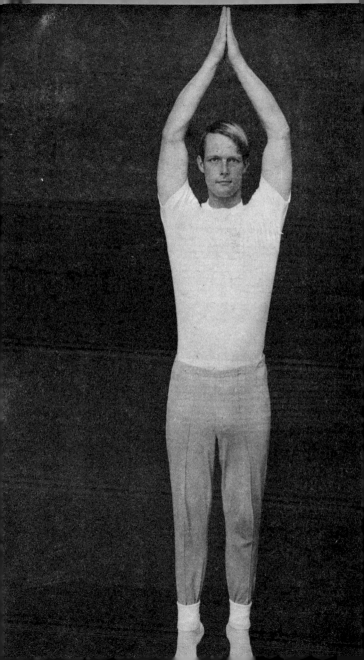

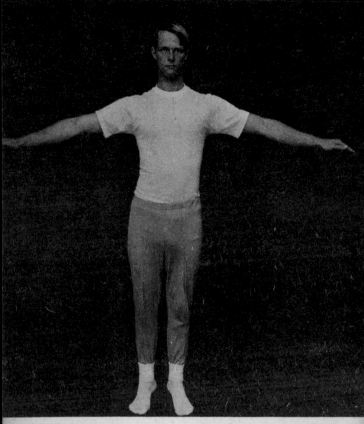

FIG. 4 *Begin to slowly exhale and lower the arms. Lower the feet partially.*

FIG. 5 *Continue the very deep exhalation. The abdomen is contracted and you allow yourself to "wither". The body assumes a limp position as the deep exhalation is completed. Without pause the inhalation and body movements are repeated.*

Perform the Complete Breath Standing three times without pause.

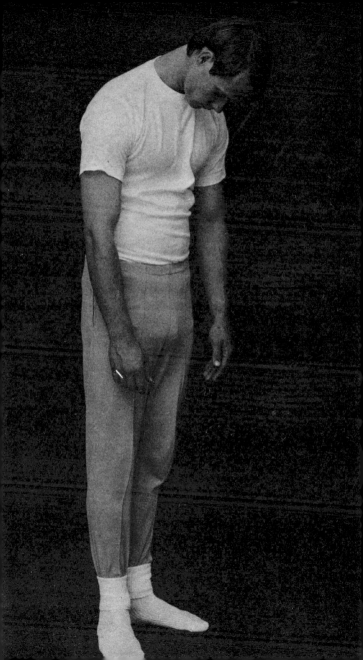

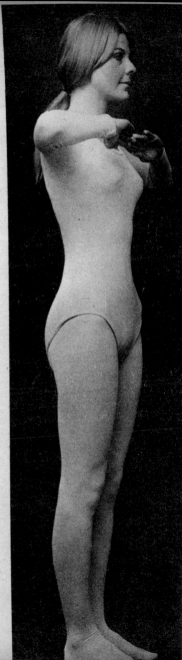

CHEST EXPANSION (Figs. 6-12)

FIG. 6 *In a standing posture gracefully raise your arms and bring your hands into the position illustrated.*

FIG. 7 *Slowly stretch your arms straight out before you. Feel the elbows stretch.*

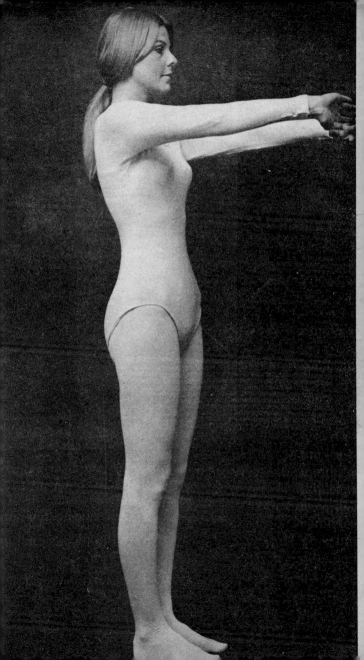

FIG. 8 *Bring your arms straight back as far as possible, in line with your shoulders. When you can go no farther, drop your arms so that you can interlace your fingers. Hold your trunk erect and do not bend forward.*

FIG. 9 *Keep your arms raised as high as possible and carefully bend backward very slowly. Do not bend your knees. When you have bent backward a moderate distance hold the position for a count of 5.*

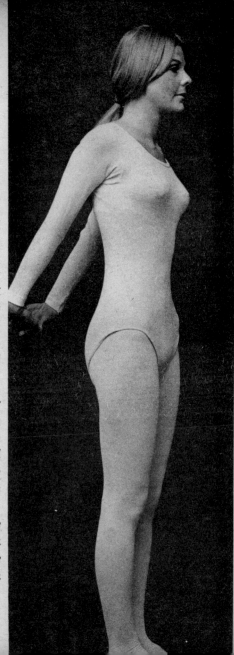

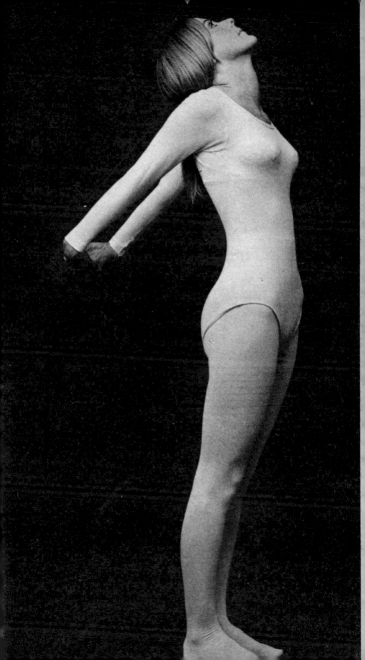

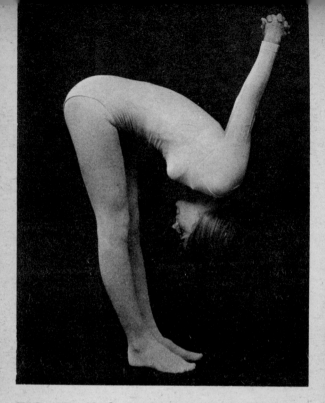

FIG. 10 *Now slowly and gently bend forward and bring your arms up and over your back. Keep the arms and legs straight. Continue to bend forward as far as possible without strain. Hold your extreme position for a count of 10.*

FIG. 11 *Straighten up slightly so that you can extend your right leg out to the side. Bend forward as before but now aim your forehead toward your right knee. Hold your extreme position for a count of 10. Bend your left knee to aid in the stretch.*

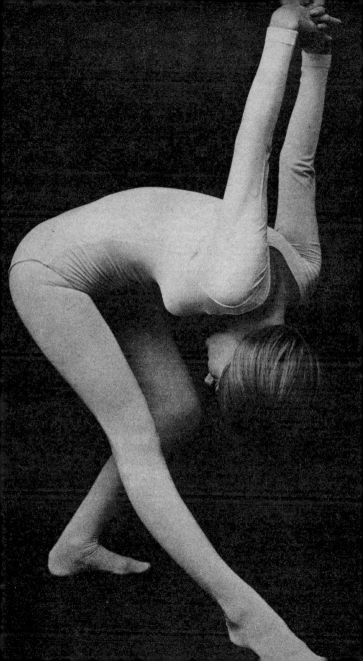

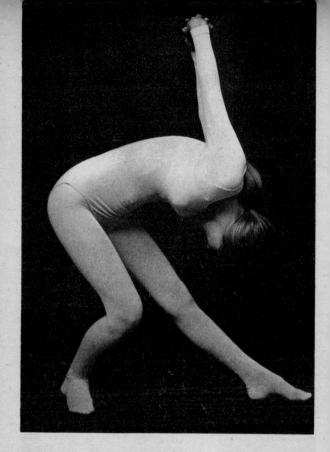

FIG. 12 *Perform the identical movements with the left leg extended. Hold your extreme position for a count of 10. When you have completed the movements straighten up very slowly and repeat the entire routine.*

Perform the Chest Expansion twice, without pause.

BACK STRETCH (Figs. 13-20)

FIG. 13 *Sit with your legs stretched straight out before you. The feet should be together. Sit erect but relaxed. Rest your hands on your knees.*

FIG. 14 *Slowly and gracefully raise your arms as illustrated.*

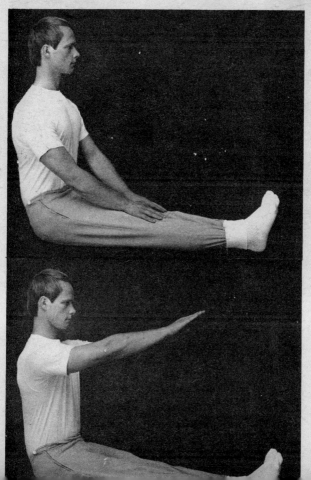

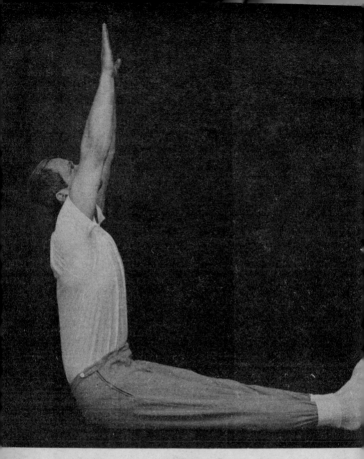

FIG. 15 *Bring your arms up to the overhead position. Look up at the hands and bend backward slightly. (This movement helps to strengthen the abdominal muscles.)*

FIG. 16 *Slowly and gracefully stretch forward and down.*

FIG. 17 *Take a firm hold on your knees or calves.*

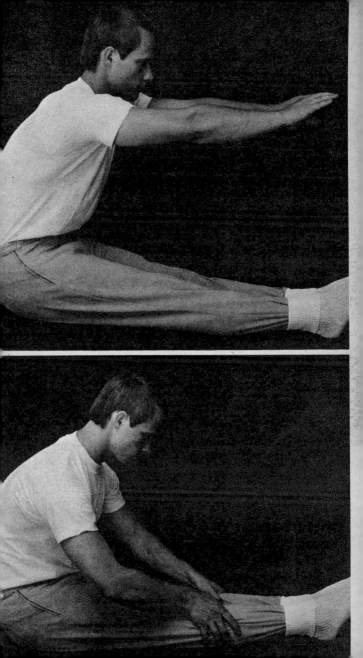

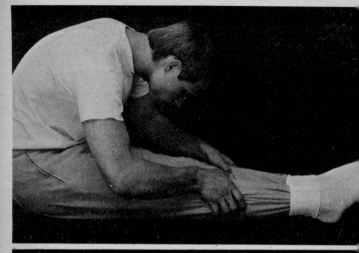

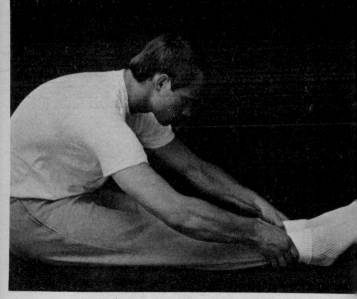

FIG. 18 *Gently pull your trunk downward as far as possible without strain. Bend your elbows outward and allow your neck to relax. Hold your extreme position without moving for a count of 5.*

FIG. 19 *Slide your hands farther down the legs and attempt to take a firm hold of the ankles.*

FIG. 20 *Pull your trunk gently downward as before, bending the elbows outward. Rest your forehead as close to your knees as possible without strain. Relax all muscles of your body. Hold the extreme position without motion for a count of 5.*

Slowly straighten up to the position of Fig. 13 and repeat both knee and ankles stretches. Perform three times in all.

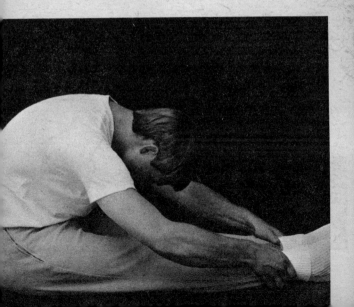

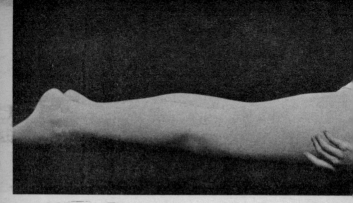

COBRA (Figs. 21-28)

FIG. 21 *Lie with your forehead resting on the floor (or on your exercise mat). Arms are at sides and the body is completely relaxed.*

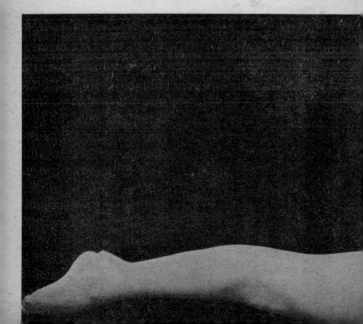

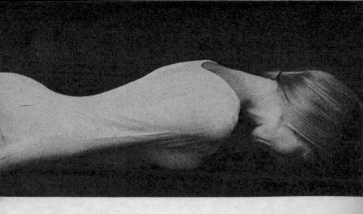

FIG. 22 *In very slow motion tilt your head back and using your back muscles raise your trunk as far from the floor as possible without the use of your hands.*

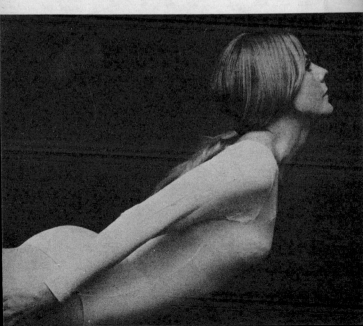

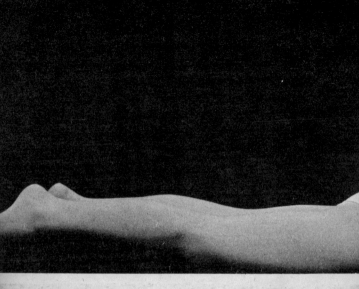

FIG. 23 *Slowly and gracefully bring your hands into the exact position illustrated— with the fingers pointing toward one another.*

FIG. 24 *Now continue to raise the trunk. This raising should be performed so slowly that you can almost feel each vertebra working out. The head tilts backward and the spine is continually arched.*

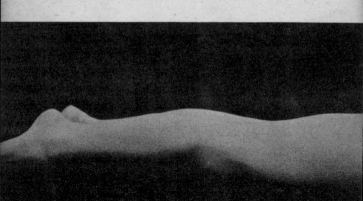

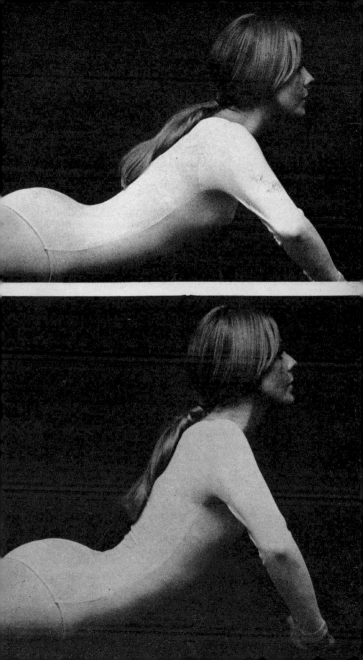

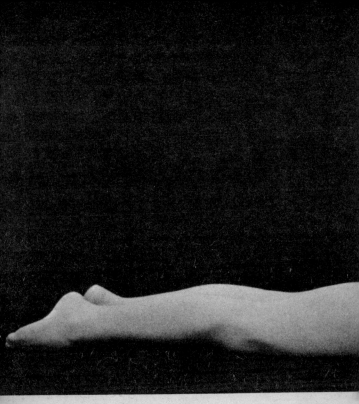

FIG. 25 *The completed posture. During initial attempts you push up only as far as you can without strain, then stop. In this extreme position, which is attained with practice, your arms are straight and your head is tilted far back. The legs are relaxed. Hold whatever extreme position you can attain for a count of 10.*

FIG. 26 *Begin to lower yourself very slowly in the exact reverse procedure. It is important to keep your spine arched as the trunk is lowered.*

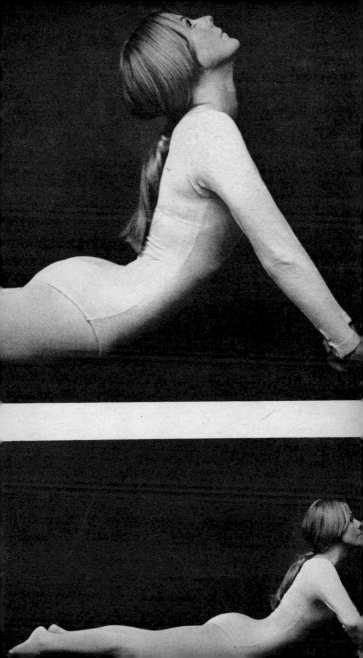

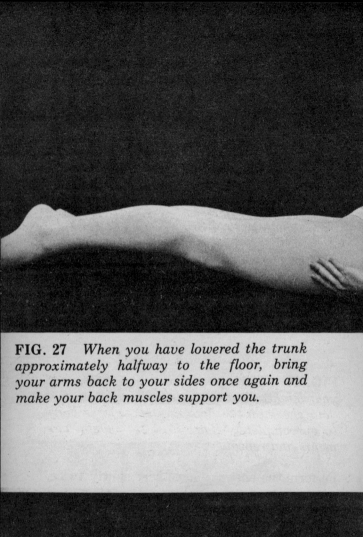

FIG. 27 *When you have lowered the trunk approximately halfway to the floor, bring your arms back to your sides once again and make your back muscles support you.*

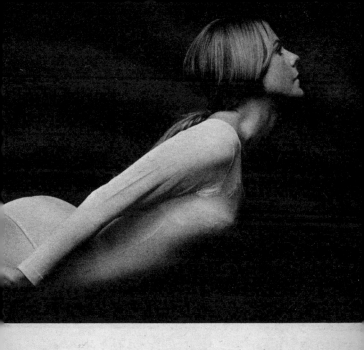

FIG. 28 *Continue to lower the trunk until your forehead touches on the floor. Then rest your cheek on the floor and allow your body to go completely limp. Rest for several moments and repeat.*

Perform the entire routine very slowly twice.

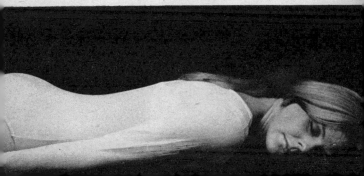

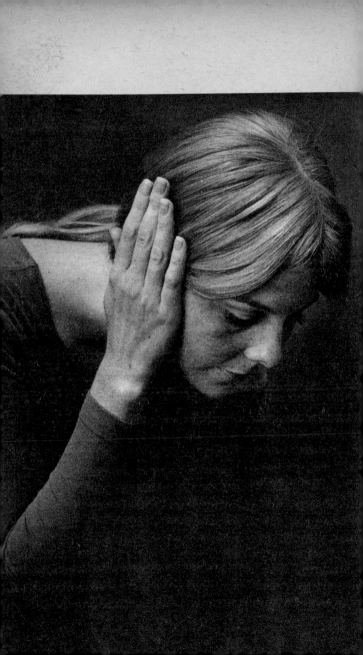

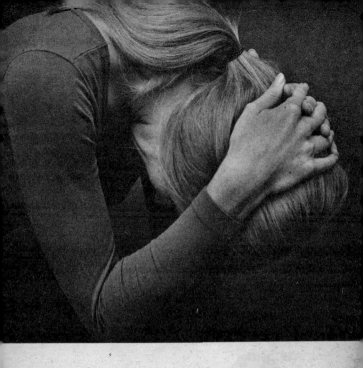

HEAD TWIST (Figs. 29-31)

FIG. 29 *Place your elbows and arms as illustrated. Your head rests between your hands.*

FIG. 30 *Clasp your hands firmly on the back of your head and gently push down until your chin touches your chest. Close your eyes. Hold for a count of 10.*

FIG. 31 *Do not move your arms. Turn your head slowly and rest your chin in your right palm. Grip the back of your head firmly with your left hand. Turn your head slowly as far as possible to your right. Keep your eyes closed. Hold your extreme position for a count of 10.*

Do not move your arms. Perform the identical movements to the left side by resting your chin in your left palm and having the right hand grip the back of your head.

Perform the Head Twist once in each of the three positions.

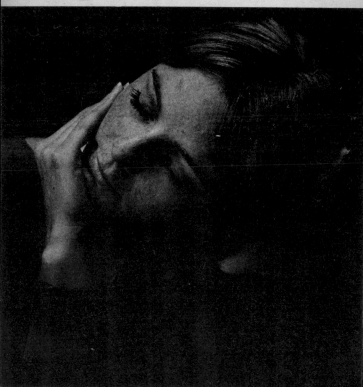

MODIFIED HEAD STAND (Figs. 32-35)

FIG. 32 *Sit on your heels; interlace your fingers as illustrated.*

FIG. 33 *Bend forward and place your hands on the floor.*

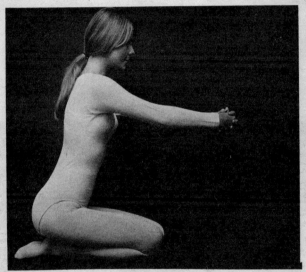

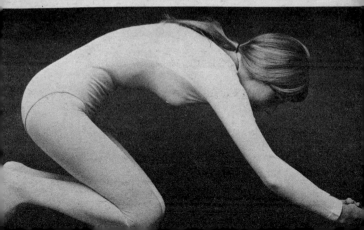

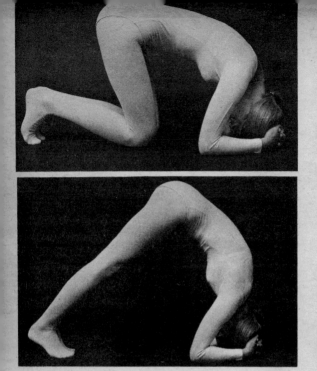

FIG. 34 *The top of your head touches the floor and the back of your head rests firmly against your locked fingers. Toes are in the position illustrated.*

FIG. 35 *Now place your full weight on the lower arms. Push down with your toes and raise the body as illustrated.*

Hold this position for 15 seconds in the beginning and gradually increase the time to 1 minute.

To come out of the posture, lower the knees to the floor and rest with the head down for an additional 15 seconds. Perform once only.

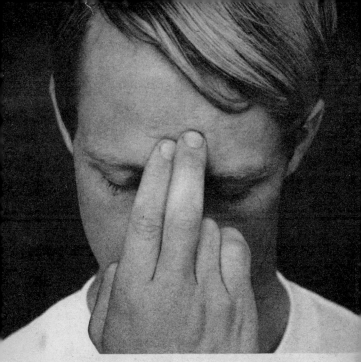

ALTERNATE NOSTRIL BREATHING
(Figs. 36-39)

FIG. 36 *Sit in a cross-legged or Lotus posture. This breathing technique is performed in three parts: inhalation, retention, exhalation. The flow of your breath is directed by stopping your nostrils alternately.*

Study the illustration and note carefully the position of the hand and fingers. Place the tip of your right thumb against your right nostril. Put your index and middle fingers together on your forehead (on the "third eye' center). Place your ring finger lightly against your left nostril. The hand remains relaxed.

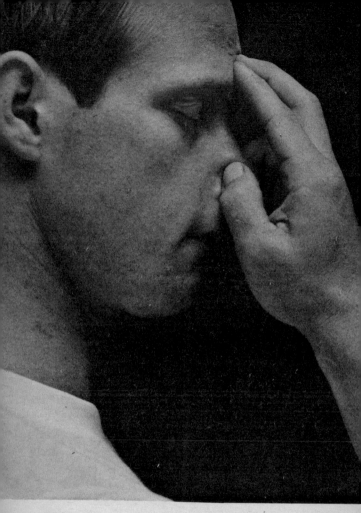

FIG. 37 *Exhale deeply through both nostrils. Now close your right nostril by pressing your thumb against it; the left nostril remains open. Inhale a slow, quiet Complete Breath through your left nostril during a rhythmic count of 8 beats.*

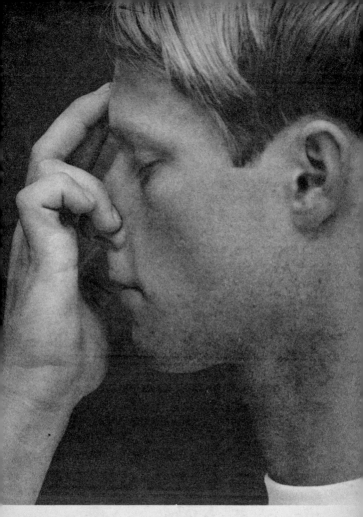

FIG. 38 *Keep the right nostril closed and now close the left nostril with the ring finger as illustrated. Both nostrils are thus tightly closed and the breath is retained in the lungs for a rhythmic count of 4.*

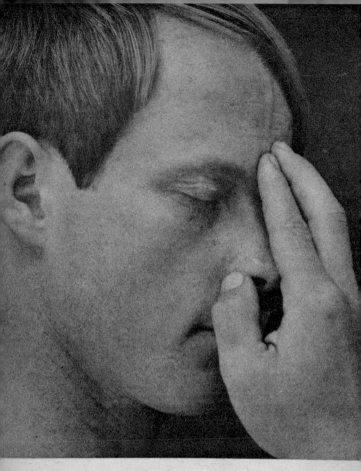

FIG. 39 *Now remove the thumb from your right nostril (keeping the left closed) and slowly and quietly exhale deeply through the right nostril during a rhythmic count of 8 beats.*

When the air is completely exhaled from your lungs during the count of 8, resume the inhalation — without missing a beat in your rhythmic counting — through your right nostril (the same nostril through which you just finished exhaling).

When the inhalation through your right nostril is completed during a rhythmic count of 8 beats, retain the air in your lungs by closing both nostrils as before. Hold for a rhythmic count of 4 beats. Then, without missing a beat, open your left nostril by removing the ring finger and exhale deeply through your left nostril during a rhythmic count of 8 beats (the right nostril remains closed). Without missing a beat in your counting begin the entire routine again by inhaling through your left nostril in a count of 8 beats, and so on.

Each time you return to the original point, that is, inhaling through your left nostril, you have completed one round of Alternate Nostril Breathing.

Summary:
    Inhale through the left....................**8 beats**
    Retain (both nostrils closed) ....**4 beats**
    Exhale through the right ....**8 beats**

    Inhale through the right ....**8 beats**
    Retain (both nostrils closed) ....**4 beats**
    Exhale through the left ....**8 beats**
    THIS COMPLETES ONE ROUND

Perform 5 rounds of Alternate Nostril Breathing. When you have completed the final round, place your right hand on your knee and remain very still for several minutes. You will experience a profound sense of serenity.

A GUIDE
TO
MEDITATION:
ACTIVE AND PASSIVE

A GUIDE TO MEDITATION PRACTICE

Since time immemorial the great masters, gurus, prophets, sages and wise men of all cultures have stressed the necessity for meditation and have taught its various methods. Although meditation is practiced in many different forms throughout the world, the ultimate objective of all forms is the same: to transcend the ordinary mind and become aware of the Universal Mind. It is in the realization of Universal Mind, as we have tried to show, that peace and fulfillment are experienced.

The meditation techniques offered in this book are, for the most part, simple. However, they will prove highly effective in pointing the way toward the ultimate objective.

The following information will help you achieve the best results from your meditation practice:

1. Make every effort to practice daily, because the effect of meditation is cumulative. Four to five times a week is an absolute must for all serious students.

2. Sunrise, sunset and before retiring are excellent times for practice. If your circumstances do not permit this, choose any time when you can be alone and

completely quiet. Ideally, you should practice at approximately the same time each day.

3. The time spent in each practice is up to the individual—the longer, the better. Ten to twenty minutes is a minimum period.

4. Select a pleasant, secluded place. It must be quiet and have good vibrations. Flowers, incense and other objects associated with meditation and peace can be placed in the meditation area if you are so inclined. This is the traditional procedure, although not essential.

5. Perform the Posture Routine of Section II exactly as directed.

6. Choose one or more of the meditation exercises and practice with them according to the directions. No more than two exercises should be used in any one practice session. Selection of the techniques is a completely personal matter governed largely by natural attraction. After making a number of preliminary experiments with *all* of the meditation exercises offered in this book, you will be able to make a decision as to which seem to be the most meaningful to you. You can then work exclusively with your selection, occasionally introducing some of the other exercises to determine whether they

have increased in value. If so, you can then include them in your practice.

Your experiences in working seriously and patiently with the chosen techniques will continually change; "insight," "growth," "expansion," "realization" are some of the words that might convey what transpires. But, as repeatedly pointed out in Section I, meditation is an *experience* and always transcends our attempts to confine it within the limits of a definition. *You can only know meditation by practicing it!*

For ease of selection and practice, we offer, in the following pages, a summary of meditation techniques outlined in Section I. These are arranged in the "active" and "passive" categories. Certain techniques are instructed in greater detail than in Section I and a number of alternate methods are offered. The additional instruction is taken from the author's record album, *Yoga Meditation*.

ACTIVE MEDITATION

1. Observation of the *body in action*. (See page 23)
2. Observation of the *ordinary mind in action*. (See page 38)
3. *Experience* as meditation. (See page 126)

PASSIVE MEDITATION

1. **CONCENTRATION WITH THE EYE**
   (a) On various objects. See page 51.
   (b) Candle Meditation

   Candle Meditation is a very ancient and highly restful practice in the art of one-pointedness—that is, being able to direct your attention fully to one point and not allowing your mind to wander.

   This exercise is performed in two parts:

   - First, gazing steadily at the flame of a candle for approximately 2 minutes.

   - Second, placing your palms over your closed eyes and attempting to retain the image of the flame for an additional 2 minutes.

   - Before you start, your candle should be lit and placed about 3-5 feet from where you are. You should be seated in the usual Lotus posture. (See page 62). Then, fix your gaze steadily on the flame. Keep your eyelids in their natural position....Blink as necessary.

- Observe now the subtle movements of the flame......
  (30 beats)*

- Continue to observe the movements of the flame......
  (30 beats)

- Now observe the various colors contained in the flame......
  (30 beats)

- Continue to observe the various colors contained within the flame......
  (30 beats)

- Now close your eyes and place your palms lightly over your lids....... Retain the image of the flame and try to center this image......
  (15 beats)

- Observe the characteristics of the flame now.....the differences in form and colors......
  (30 beats)

- If the flame disappears, you can bring it back....simply by willing it back...
  (30 beats)

---

* *Each beat represents approximately one second. After repeated performance of these meditations, you'll find you will no longer have to refer to the text for either instruction or time intervals.*

- As the image begins to fade, continue to observe the subtle changes in form and color as it fades......
  (30 beats)

- Now return your hands to your knees and open your eyes. You may repeat this exercise if you wish.

2. CONCENTRATION WITH THE EAR
See page 69.

3. CONCENTRATION WITH THE BREATH

The following technique is offered as an alternative to that given on page 78. Both are equally effective.

- This meditation is performed with your breathing. First, you must focus your full attention on the way in which you breathe, and then establish a rhythm for the breathing. You should be seated comfortably but firmly in the recommended posture, with your head straight and your eyelids partially lowered. Be relaxed...Now observe your breathing. It should be low breathing—that is, movement occurs only in the abdominal area. With each inhalation, push the abdomen out slightly and mentally direct the air into the abdominal area. Do this easily... without effort.

- Now, attempt to slow the rhythm of your breathing.....

    (6 beats)

- Breathe as silently as possible....

    (6 beats)

- Now you are sitting correctly, breathing silently and slowly, and performing a slight abdominal movement each time you inhale....

- The next step is to establish a rhythm for your breathing. Count 2 for inhaling.. 2 for exhaling....and then rest without breathing for a count of 2.

- Now follow this rhythm. Begin to inhale: 1, 2....exhale, 1, 2.... rest, 1, 2. Inhale, 2....exhale, 2.... rest, 2. Inhale, 2....exhale, 2....rest, 2. Continue this rhythm by yourself. Inhale, 2....exhale, 2....rest, 2. Inhale, 2....exhale, 2.... rest, 2. Inhale, 2....exhale, 2....rest, 2.

- Now you must count your breath and focus your full attention on the counting. Each rest between breaths will count as one complete round....and you will count silently to 10 complete rounds. You must keep your attention concentrated or you will lose the count. Ready... Begin:

- Inhale, 2....exhale, 2....rest, 2. Round

2: inhale, 2....exhale, 2....rest, 2. Round
3: inhale, 2....exhale, 2....rest, 2. Round
4: Continue by yourself in the same
rhythm. Round 5....Round 6....Do
not allow your attention to wander
....Round 7....Round 8....Remember,
don't allow your attention to wander....
Round 9....Round 10....rest.

- When you have finished 10 rounds,
  you may continue this exercise for
  several more groups of 10 as you wish.

4. CONCENTRATION WITH THE VOICE

In this exercise, you meditate with the
voice. You will be using a very ancient Sanskrit syllable which has been chanted by millions of persons throughout the centuries to
experience a profound sense of peace.

The sound, as you know from Chapter 6, is
composed of two letters—O and M. To make
the sound *OM* (as in "home"), hold the O for
5 beats...O-O-O-O-O. And then hold a resonant M sound for 5 beats...M-M-M-M-M.
Then take a Deep Complete Breath in 5 beats
for the next repetition.

The voice is medium-loud and steady.
The sound should come from the abdomen,
not the chest. The M sound is extremely
resonant and should be made to vibrate
strongly.

- Sit in the recommended posture. Now

perform the chanting....Hold your attention steadfastly on the sound of your own voice. Do not let your attention wander....

- Let us begin by taking a Deep Complete Breath to a count of 5 beats. Exhale completely. Breathe 1...2...3...4... 5... O-O-O-O-O ... M-M-M-M-M. Inhale 1...2...3...4...5...O-O-O-O-O ...M-M-M-M-M. Inhale 1...2... 3... 4... 5... O-O-O-O-O ... M-M-M-M-M. Deep Complete Breath 1... 2...3... 4...5... O-O-O-O-O... M-M-M-M-M... and so forth.

Throughout the chanting, hold your attention steadfastly on the sound of your voice. Do not allow your attention to wander.

- Begin, once again, by taking a Deep Complete Breath for a count of 5 beats, exhale completely, then....O-O-O-O-O...M-M-M-M-M...inhale and repeat ... O-O-O-O-O... M-M-M-M-M.... inhale and repeat...O-O-O-O-O...M-M-M-M-M...inhale and repeat....O-O-O-O-O...M-M-M-M-M...inhale and repeat ... O-O-O-O-O ... M-M-M-M-M ... Rest.

- Repeat each OM sound as many times as you wish.

5. DIRECTING THE LIFE FORCE. See
page 105.

6. DEEP RELAXATION

The objective of this meditation technique
is to achieve deep relaxation through awareness of the body.

- First, sit in the Half or Full Lotus
  position. To do the Full Lotus (the clas-
  sic meditation and relaxation position),
  place the left foot as high on the right
  thigh as you can. If the left foot can
  touch the floor without straining, you
  should now try placing the right foot
  on the left thigh. In the Half Lotus,
  you place your right foot so that it is
  resting against the upper part of the
  left thigh (the left foot is outstretched).
  Then you place the left foot so that it
  is in the fold of the right leg. It is probably easier on your legs than the Full
  Lotus. With forefinger against the
  thumb, rest both hands on knees or on
  the floor behind you. If either of these
  two positions is too difficult for you
  (even after practice), a simple cross-legged posture will do. Also see page 153.

- You can do Deep Relaxation whenever
  you need quick relief from tension

Become very aware of and relax the following parts of your body....in this order...

- Relax completely your right foot ... calf...thigh...Then your left foot ... calf...thigh.

- Relax the abdomen....

- Remain sitting erect but relax the base of the spine....the lower back.... the upper back.

- Relax the shoulders, but don't slump.

- Keep the correct position of your fingers, but relax your right hand...forearm...upper arm. Your left hand... forearm...upper arm.

- Relax the muscles of your face.

- Now you can determine if you have entirely relaxed each of these areas by becoming very aware of them once more.

- Relax completely your right foot... calf...thigh. Your left foot...calf... thigh. Your abdomen.

- Remain sitting erect but relax the base of the spine...lower back...upper back.

- Relax the shoulders, but don't slump.

- Keep the position of your fingers but relax your right hand...hand...forearm ...upper arm. Left hand...forearm ...upper arm,

- Relax the muscles of your face.

- Now your entire organism is deeply relaxed and yet you are fully aware.... Feel this state of quiet awareness....

7. MEDITATION ON THE QUESTION: "WHO AM I?" See page 112

8. MEDITATION WITHOUT SEED

A more advanced and highly revealing form of meditation is Meditation Without Seed. Here, you will rest the mind by literally shutting it off and not permitting any thought whatsoever to enter.

With this technique, you will learn a great deal about the continual turmoil of the mind and the importance of being able to rest it.

- This form of meditation should take about 3 minutes. During this interval, whenever you observe that you are being distracted by a thought, you must cast it gently but firmly aside and keep your mind empty.

- Because you hold on to nothing whatsoever, this practice is called Meditation Without Seed.

- First, empty your mind of all thoughts and distractions and become aware of what occurs if you stop thinking in your usual manner.....

  (60 beats)

- Keep your mind empty.....

  (60 beats)

- Be aware of what it is like to have stopped thinking.....

  (60 beats)

- Now 3 minutes have passed. You may now continue this exercise further if you wish.

YOGA FOR HEALTH,
Mr. Hittleman's television series, may
be seen in many areas. For a free newsletter
and catalog containing the author's
other publications and information regarding
his Meditation Album, write to:
Richard Hittleman,
P.O. Box 475
Carmel, California
93921